Introduction to Dietetic Practice

Introduction to Dietetic Practice

Katie Ferraro, MPH, RD, CDE

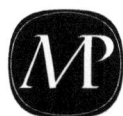

MOMENTUM PRESS
HEALTH

Introduction to Dietetic Practice

First published in 2016 by
Momentum Press, LLC
222 East 46th Street, New York, NY 10017
www.momentumpress.net

ISBN-13: 978-1-60650-721-6 (print)
ISBN-13: 978-1-60650-722-3 (e-book)

Momentum Press Nutrition and Dietetics Practice Collection

DOI: 10.5643/9781606507223

Cover and interior design by S4Carlisle Publishing Services Private Ltd., Chennai, India

First edition: 2016

10 9 8 7 6 5 4 3 2 1

Printed in the United States of America.

Abstract

Introduction to Dietetic Practice focuses on the core principles of dietetic practice and introduces readers to advancements and opportunities in the field. The content includes an overview of the profession as it exists today, a summary of the history of dietetics in North America, a review of nutrition credential and educational pathways, career opportunities in the field, and a look at the future need for credentialed nutrition and dietetics professionals.

Keywords

Registered Dietitian, nutritionist, nutrition, nutrition jobs, dietetics, clinical nutrition, community nutrition, sports nutrition, lifecycle nutrition, diet therapy, medical nutrition therapy

Contents

List of Tables

CHAPTER 1

Overview of the Profession of Nutrition and Dietetics

Chapter Abstract

Dietetics refers to the science and art of applying the principles of food and nutrition to health (AND, 2015d). As a profession, nutrition and dietetics is a vast and expanding field, essentially encompassing and affecting any environment where food choices are being made and health outcomes are being determined. This chapter seeks to provide an overview of the profession of nutrition and dietetics, analyzing the need for credentialed professionals and evaluating the impact that evidence-based dietary guidance can have on individual, group, and institutional populations. The reader will be introduced to the rationale for nutrition education, data supporting its inclusion as a part of a comprehensive health care plan, tips for effective counseling and program planning as well as the impact of community-based approaches to combatting overweight and obesity, and reducing chronic disease risk.

Introduction to Dietetic Practice

It is often said, "You are what you eat." As a population, the way we are eating is clearly *not* working. In the United States, 69 percent of adults are overweight or obese (CDC, 2015a) and the dietary decisions that are made—or not made—over the course of one's lifetime take a serious toll on health. A close analysis of the leading causes of death in the United States reveals that four of the top ten leading causes of death—heart disease, diabetes, stroke, and cancer—are strongly linked to diet (CDC, 2015a), (HHS, 2001).

Unfortunately, these poor health outcomes are not just limited to adult populations; in fact, due to rising rates of obesity, it is thought that this may be the first generation of children who have shorter life spans than their parents (Olshansky et al., 2005). Chronic diseases previously seen only in the later stages of life are now afflicting younger patients due almost solely to the impact of overweight and obesity. Today, 20.5 percent of adolescents aged 12 to 19, 17.7 percent of children aged 6 to 11, and 8.4 percent of children aged 2 to 5 are clinically obese (CDC, 2015). Compare that to the early 1970s when just 6 percent, 4 percent, and 5 percent obesity rates were seen in those respective age groups (Ogden, Flegal, Carroll, & Johnson, 2002).

While there is certainly a disagreement as to whether poor diet or lack of activity is *more* responsible for expanding waistlines, most experts agree that overweight and obesity *both* contribute to increased risk of chronic disease. With regard to diet, we are surrounded by a 24-hour food environment where continuous access to cheap, empty calories fuels constant eating. In fact, the average number of daily calories available to each person in the United States increased by 600 calories from 1970 to 2008 (U.S. Department of Agriculture, Economic Research Service, 2014). When it comes to exertion, only one-quarter of U.S. children and youth aged 6 to 15 meet the recommendation in *Physical Activity Guidelines for Americans* to achieve at least 60 minutes of moderate to vigorous physical activity per day (HHS, 2008), (Troiano, Berrigan, Dodd, Masse, Tilert, & McDowell, 2008). Less than half (48 percent) of all adults meet the 2008 guideline recommendations for at least 2.5 hours (150 minutes) per week of physical activity (Centers for Disease Control and Prevention, 2014).

Despite these seemingly bleak statistics, this is certainly an exciting time to be working in or pursuing a career in nutrition and dietetics. Consumers are spending billions of dollars each year on weight-loss products, the public is clamoring for nutrition information about restaurant meals, the nutrition facts panel is being overhauled to improve usefulness and reflect research, and forthcoming nutrition guidelines based on research are changing the way we look at and educate populations about important topics like dietary fat and the benefits of plant-based diets. Undoubtedly, there is a heightened interest in nutrition and health as these factors drive health decisions; but when it comes to addressing the impact of poor dietary choices and physical inactivity, there is certainly much work for dietetics practitioners to do.

In the Food Marketing Institute's report *Shopping for Health*, 33 percent of respondents said they put a lot of effort into healthy eating but most (62 percent) feel improving or changing eating habits is too difficult (Food Marketing Institute, 2014). But the cumulative effect of these individual struggles is great. In their report *The State of Obesity: Better Policies for a Healthier America*, public health professionals and economists from the Trust for America's Health and the Robert Wood Johnson Foundation estimate that obesity costs in the United States range from $147 billion to $210 billion. Absenteeism from work associated with obesity costs employers $4.3 billion per year, or roughly a $506 cost to employer per obese worker per year (Trust for America's Health and the Robert Wood Johnson Foundation, 2015). Obese adults utilize a disproportionate share of our limited health care resources. An obese adult results in a 42 percent greater expenditure on direct health care costs than adults who are in a healthy weight range (Finkelstein, Trogdon, Cohen, & Dietz, 2009).

While consumers may believe that they are well informed about nutrition, these statistics clearly tell a different story. According to nutrition education expert and author Isabel Contento, individuals, groups, organizations, and institutions working in the field of nutrition and dietetics are collectively tasked to help improve overall nutrition status through the dissemination of information, facilitation of behaviors conducive to health, while also focusing on environmental change (Contento, 2011). Contento maintains that people and their environment are closely interrelated. In some cases, people may have the knowledge and/or skills required to make recommended changes, whereas others may have individual motivation, but may lack environmental support.

From a big picture standpoint, there is no shortage of opportunity or need for individuals to enter the profession of nutrition and dietetics. Whether working as educators, practitioners, researchers, or policy makers, the fact that all humans need to eat—and that our food and beverages choices ultimately drive health outcomes—provides a vast array of prospects for enacting improvements and implementing change.

Professional Nutrition Associations

A very useful place to begin the study of any profession is to research the professional associations related to that field. Professional associations conduct advocacy work, provide education and networking opportunities, and provide collaborative oversight for like-minded professionals.

Academy of Nutrition and Dietetics

In the professional practice of nutrition, the most widely recognized national credential is the registered dietitian (RD), also called registered dietitian nutritionist (RDN) credential (these credentials are covered in depth in Chapter 3). The Academy of Nutrition and Dietetics (AND, formerly called the American Dietetic Association) is the world's largest organization of food and nutrition professionals, currently claiming over 75,000 members. Members include students, RDNs, dietetic technicians, registered (DTRs), and other dietetics professionals who hold undergraduate and advanced degrees in nutrition and dietetics. The Academy "is committed to improving the nation's health and advancing the profession of dietetics through research, education and advocacy" (AND, 2015b).

The academy was originally founded as the American Dietetic Association in Cleveland, Ohio in 1917 by a group of women who collaborated to assist the government in food conservation efforts while at the same time working to improve the public's health and nutrition during the World War I era. In January 2012, the association changed its name to the Academy of Nutrition and Dietetics—a move that "complemented the focus of the organization to improve nutritional well-being, communicating the expertise of its members who are a part of a food- and science-based profession." The AND's vision is "Optimizing health through food and nutrition" and their mission is "Empowering members to be food and nutrition leaders" (AND, 2015c).

In addition to membership in the overarching association, AND members may also choose to belong to smaller subsets within the association known as dietetic practice groups (DPGs). DPGs are professional-interest groups made up of members who wish to connect with other members within their areas of interest and/or expertise. Table 1.1 contains a list of the current dietetic practice groups.

Table 1.1 American Dietetic Association dietetic practice groups (DPGs) (AND, 2015e)

Academy of Nutrition and Dietetics Dietetic Practice Groups (DPGs)
Behavioral Health Nutrition DPG
Clinical Nutrition Management DPG
Diabetes Care and Education (DCE) DPG
Dietetic Technicians in Practice DPG
Dietetics in Health Care Communities DPG
Dietitians in Business and Communications (DBC) DPG
Dietitians in Integrative and Functional Medicine DPG
Dietitians in Nutrition Support (DNS) DPG
Food and Culinary Professionals DPG
Healthy Aging DPG
Hunger and Environmental Nutrition DPG
Management in Food and Nutrition Systems DPG
Medical Nutrition Practice Group DPG
Nutrition Education for the Public (NEP) DPG
Nutrition Educators of Health Professionals (NEHP) DPG
Nutrition Entrepreneurs (NE) DPG
Oncology Nutrition DPG
Pediatric Nutrition DPG
Public Health / Community Nutrition DPG
Renal Dietitians DPG
Research DPG
School Nutrition Services DPG
Sports, Cardiovascular and Wellness Nutrition DPG
Vegetarian Nutrition DPG
Weight Management DPG
Women's Health DPG

Table 1.2 American Dietetic Association member interest groups (MIGs) (AND, 2015f)

Academy of Nutrition and Dietetics Member Interest Groups (MIGs)
Asian Indians in Nutrition and Dietetics (AIND)
Chinese Americans in Dietetics and Nutrition (CADN)
Fifty Plus in Nutrition and Dietetics (FPIND)
Filipino Americans in Dietetics and Nutrition (FADAN)
Jewish Member Interest Group (JMIG)
Latinos and Hispanics in Dietetics and Nutrition (LAHIDAN)
Muslims in Dietetics and Nutrition (MIDAN)
National Organization of Blacks in Dietetics and Nutrition (NOBIDAN)
National Organization of Men in Nutrition (NOMIN)
Thirty and Under in Nutrition and Dietetics (TUND)

In addition to the dietetic practice groups, AND members may also choose to identify with member interest groups (MIGs). Member interest groups are groups of Academy members who share a common interest. Unlike the DPGs, MIGs focus on areas other than practice or geographic location; they reflect the many characteristics of the AND's membership and the public it serves. Table 1.2 lists the AND's member interest groups.

Accreditation Council for Education in Nutrition and Dietetics (ACEND)

The Accreditation Council for Education in Nutrition and Dietetics (ACEND®) is the Academy of Nutrition and Dietetics' accrediting agency for education programs that prepare students for careers as registered dietitian nutritionists or dietetic technicians, registered (DTRs) (AND, 2015). ACEND was formerly known as the Commission on Accreditation for Dietetics Education (CADE) and it essentially serves as the accrediting agency for the Academy of Nutrition and Dietetics. Programs that meet accreditation standards are accredited by ACEND.

ACEND's mission includes serving the public "by establishing and enforcing eligibility requirements and accreditation standards that ensure the quality and continued improvement of nutrition and dietetics education programs that reflect the evolving practice of dietetics" (AND, 2015a). Students and future practitioners who are interested in studying to become a registered dietitian nutrition or dietetic technician, registered are encouraged to visit the ACEND website to explore accredited education programs. Available programs include coordinated programs in dietetics, didactic programs in dietetics, dietetic internships and dietetic technician programs. More information about the various tracts available for interested future professionals is contained in Chapter 3. To view the ACEND accredited dietetics education programs, visit http://www.eatrightacend.org/ACEND/content.aspx?id=6442485414.

Society for Nutrition Education and Behavior

The Society for Nutrition Education and Behavior (SNEB) represents the unique professional interests of nutrition educators in the United States and worldwide (Society for Nutrition Education and Behavior, 2014). The association seeks to promote effective nutrition education and healthy behaviors through the avenues of research and policy and practice. Members include professionals who work in nutrition education and health promotion. This may include universities and schools, government agencies, cooperative extension, communications and public relations firms, the food industry, voluntary and service organizations, and other areas where reliable nutrition and health information are disseminated. Table 1.3 outlines the vision, mission, and goals of SNEB. To learn more, visit the SNEB website at www.sneb.org.

The Case for Medical Nutrition Therapy

If you do decide, or have already decided, to devote yourself to the practice of nutrition and dietetics, you are likely curious to know what approaches have been "proven" to work. Take a brief tour of the internet, searching for phrases like "pound shedding diet", "proven weight loss cleanse," and "ancient remedy supplements" and you're likely to come

Table 1.3 The vision, mission, and goals of the Society for Nutrition Education and Behavior (SNEB) (Society for Nutrition Education and Behavior, 2014)

The Society for Nutrition Education and Behavior (SNEB) Vision
Healthy communities, food systems and behaviors
SNEB Mission
To promote effective nutrition education and healthy behavior through research, policy and practice
SNEB Goals
Grow and maintain a dynamic society, serving nutrition educators around the world
Support the effective practice of nutrition education
Advocate for policies that support healthy communities, food systems, and behaviors
Promote research related to effective nutrition education and behavior change at the individual, community and policy levels
Build collaborations with organizations, industries, and government to promote healthy communities, food systems, and behaviors

across an endless stream of ineffective therapies, potentially dangerous supplements, and innumerable lotions and potions all promising the latest and greatest in weight loss, health improvement, or miraculous recoveries that for the most part do *not* work. So what then is the antidote? The answer is Medical Nutrition Therapy (MNT). MNT refers to the therapeutic approach to treating and preventing disease through implementation of food and nutrition interventions. MNT provided by a registered dietitian nutritionist may include:

- Review of current intake patterns
- Thorough assessment of nutritional health
- Individualized nutrition treatment plan (AND, 2014)

In today's medical and reimbursement environment, outcomes matter—and as such, it is important that nutrition professionals can prove the efficacy of their interventions and treatment plans. MNT provided by an RDN has been demonstrated to be an effective approach to managing diabetes, hypertension, disorders of lipid metabolism, HIV infection, pregnancy, chronic kidney disease, and unintended weight loss in older adults (AND, 2013).

With overweight and obesity reaching new and staggering rates, it is important that credentialed professionals demonstrate the effectiveness of their practice. The effectiveness of MNT with an RD is further demonstrated in improved outcomes related to weight management:

- MNT provided by an RD for overweight and obese adults for less than 6 months yields significant weight losses of approximately 1 to 2 pounds per week.
- MNT for 6 to 12 months yielded significant mean weight losses of up to 10 percent of body weight with maintenance of this weight loss beyond 1 year.
- Overweight and obese people who received MNT provided by an RD, in addition to an obesity-related health management program that included physician visits, nursing support, and educational materials and tolls, were more likely to achieve clinically significant weight loss than individuals who did not receive MNT (AND, 2013).

From a financial standpoint, MNT provided by the RD for two conditions—diabetes and non-dialysis kidney disease—is a covered, billable benefit by Medicare Part B and some other private health insurance companies. According to one analysis, for every dollar invested in the RD-led lifestyle modification program, there was a demonstrated return of $14.58 (Wolf, Crowther, Nadler, & Bovbjerg, 2009).

Nutrition Education and Counseling in Practice

While spending patterns, records of internet searches, and discussions with friends and colleagues indicate that the typical American may be *interested* in nutrition, consumption patterns, inactivity levels, and obesity rates reveal that most people are not actually putting this knowledge into practice. Informing individuals and groups about healthful practices may be one thing, but helping them translate that information into action is an entirely different undertaking. Nutrition practitioners are at their core educators, and nutrition educators work on the frontlines of enacting individual and community-level changes.

Addressing Dietary Intake Using Food Records

Whether a nutrition practitioner is working in a face-to-face counseling environment, on a population-based dietary research study, or in a community or institutional setting, he or she will benefit from a basic understanding of dietary assessment. The availability of dietary assessment and nutrient analysis tools range from the very simple to the incredibly complex.

24-Hour Recall

The 24-hour recall is considered to be among the most commonly used dietary intake screening tools (Lee & Nieman, 2007). The basic premise of the 24-hour recall is that a well-trained interviewer quickly elicits important patient nutrition and health data based on reported food and beverage intake patterns. When subjected to the 24-hour recall method, the respondent is questioned in detail regarding all of the food and drink he or she consumed in the preceding 24 hours. The interviewer probes for additional information regarding food preparation methods, portion sizes, physical location of eating events, and may even ask questions about emotions and feelings associated with the intake.

Food Records and Food Diaries

Other methods of rapid dietary intake include the use of food records or food diaries. These are logs kept by the respondent that are brought to the practitioner for review. Nutrition practitioners or educators may request that a new patient or client fill out a food record form or keep a food diary or journal for a prescribed number of days and bring that completed record to the initial appointment. While any variation of total days worth of food records may be requested (e.g., one, three, or five days), many practitioners find it helpful to request and review three days of intake: two weekdays and one weekend day (accounting for the fact that most individuals eat, drink, and behave differently on the weekend compared to the weekdays).

Once the completed records have been received, the practitioner reviews intake and will likely then perform any one of a number of analyses to identify possible areas of under- or overnutrition. Even without the assistance of detailed electronic nutrient analysis, a quick review of a patient's three-day food record can be very telling, and it often sets the stage for the ensuing conversation regarding diet. Does the patient regularly skip meals? Why? Does the typical day's intake appear to feature all white- and brown-colored foods? Are the majority of meals coming from a fast food outlet or restaurant location? Do the stated portion sizes reflect realistic intake levels? Food records of course do not tell the whole story, but they are an important starting point for the practitioner to develop rapport with the client and to gain valuable insight into current eating patterns.

As with all record keeping, there are inherent limitations to self-kept records. These may include under-reporting in areas such as binge eating and alcohol consumption or over-reporting of foods perceived to be healthy (Lee & Nieman, 2007). Due to time constraints in the initial screening period, brief dietary intake assessment methods like the 24-hour dietary recall or quick questioning about diet history may be preferred over more thorough and lengthy methods. There are validated nutrition screeners that practitioners can access to employ in their individual practice and these will be discussed later in the chapter.

Food Frequency

Food frequency tools such as a Food Frequency Questionnaire (FFQ) employ a retrospective approach to quantify how often during a set period of time (e.g., day, week, month, or year) a type of food or food group is consumed. FFQs are used commonly in large epidemiologic studies that explore the link between diet and health as well as in national household-level surveys such as the National Health and Nutrition Examination Survey (NHANES). FFQs can also be tailored for use in the clinic, office, or community setting, and they can be configured to probe for information about certain nutrients or dietary components (e.g., calcium, caffeine, soy, or fiber intake). The foods in an FFQ are grouped together because of similar nutrient profiles. The respondent answers questions about how frequently certain foods or types of foods are consumed and the results are then either scanned or coded to reveal dietary intake patterns. When compared to other dietary intake assessment methods, FFQs are relatively cost-effective, easy to complete, and require minimal oversight since they can be completed without an accompanying note taker. As with all dietary assessment methods, there are limitations, including errors in self-reporting and self-recall, as well as inevitable shifts in consumption during injury and illness that may not always be representative of usual, healthy intake.

Calorie Counts

Calorie counts are used to track actual caloric intake in an institutionalized setting. They may be requested in the inpatient or long-term care environment and require cooperation from and participation of multiple disciplines. Calorie counts are usually recorded for three days, and they are used to determine whether a patient or resident is meeting his or her estimated nutrition needs with oral intake. The means by which calories are recorded varies by institution, but generally, nursing assistants observe and document the total amount or percentages of foods and beverages consumed at each meal and snack for three days. The trained nutrition professional analyzes the recorded intake and equates that to calories per day based on known quantities of foods served in the institution. A three-day calorie intake average is determined, and the medical team then analyzes if nutrient goals are being met. Calorie counts are helpful for justifying which patients or residents may benefit from enteral nutrition or for weaning those who are receiving enteral nutrition off of tube feeding and back on to p.o. meals.

SuperTracker

The USDA's SuperTracker is a free, web-based program that helps individuals plan, track, and analyze dietary intake and physical activity. SuperTracker allows users to search and compare foods, track foods and compare them to nutrition targets, record physical activity and track progress, manage weight, set food- and beverage-related goals, and use reports to follow progress over time. The food, nutrient, and activity goals and materials in SuperTracker are aligned with the Dietary Guidelines for Americans, and the program provides personalized nutrition and physical activity plans for users. While the web-based aspects of SuperTracker contribute to its robust capabilities, it may also be a drawback for those patients, clients, or clinical settings with limited Internet access. Learn more about SuperTracker at https://www.supertracker.usda.gov.

Estimating Energy Needs

Nutrition professionals continually face situations where individual or community nutrient intake does not match nutrient needs. Much of the increased risk of chronic disease and rising burden of overweight and obesity can be attributable to excessive calorie intake. Nutrition practitioners can help clients and communities more closely match their energy (calorie) needs by first estimating patients' energy needs and educating them about the same. Estimating a patient's energy (or total caloric) needs can be accomplished through the use of equipment, or in the absence of such equipment, predictive equations. The metabolic cart is considered to be the most accurate means of estimating energy needs. Metabolic carts are found in research laboratories or in sophisticated medical clinics and hospitals, and they perform indirect calorimetry, the gold standard for estimating resting energy requirements. During indirect calorimetry, a metabolic cart measures the amount of heat energy produced by an individual by determining the amount of oxygen consumed and quantity of carbon dioxide eliminated. Because the equipment required to perform indirect calorimetry is costly and not widely available in all health care settings, predictive equations have been developed to help estimate energy expenditure and to calculate energy needs. The predictive equations covered in the next section are used for the adult population and are not appropriate for pregnant women or children.

Harris-Benedict Equation

The Harris-Benedict equation has historically been the most widely used equation for estimating energy requirements. It determines resting metabolic rate (RMR) that is then multiplied by an activity factor (AF) and injury factor (IF). Harris-Benedict has been found to predict RMR within 10 percent of measured RMR in 69 percent of individuals. If not entirely accurate—which no predictive equation is—the Harris-Benedict is significantly more likely to overestimate energy needs (27 percent of the time) than it is to underestimate (4 percent) (AND, 2007). The Harris-Benedict equation is as follows (where weight (W) is in kilograms, height (H) is in centimeters, and age (A) is in years):

- Men: Resting metabolic rate (RMR) = 66.47 + 13.75 × W + 5 × H – 6.76 × A
- Women: RMR = 655.1 + 9.56 × W + 1.7 × H – 4.7 × A

Mifflin-St. Jeor Equation

According to an evidence analysis conducted by the Academy of Nutrition and Dietetics, "the Mifflin-St. Jeor equation was found to be the most reliable, predicting REE within 10 percent of measured in more nonobese and obese individuals than any other equation." It was also found to have the most narrow error range (AND, 2009). The Mifflin-St. Jeor equation is as follows (where weight is in kilograms and height in centimeters):

- Men: RMR = 9.99 × weight + 6.25 × height – 4.92 × age + 5
- Women: RMR = 9.99 × weight + 6.25 × height – 4.92 × age – 161

Calories per kilogram Estimation Method

Another method of estimating energy needs is based on using a set number of calories per kilogram of body weight. The calories per kilogram method, although not scientifically validated, produces results that are close to those of the validated equations above in an easier-to-use format. The calories per kilogram method is outlined in Table 1.4 and states that:

- in order to maintain weight, multiply body weight by 25 to 30 calories per kilogram of body weight;

- to gain weight, multiply body weight by 30 to 35 calories per kilogram of body weight; and
- to lose weight, multiply body weight by 20 to 25 calories per kilogram of body weight.

Depending upon activity level and starting body weight, especially in the very overweight and obese, this ratio of calories to kilogram of body weight method may not produce entirely accurate results. It is, however, a good starting point for estimating calorie needs, which are often quite different than what the individual is actually eating. For individuals at greater than 125 percent of their ideal body weight, some practitioners use an adjusted body weight (ABW) to obtain a lower weight from which to estimate caloric needs. The adjusted body weight also has not been validated as an accurate measure, yet it is widely used in practice. The equation for determining adjusted body weight is listed in Table 1.5. For individuals at greater than 125 percent of body weight, first obtain ABW in kilograms and then multiply by 20 to 25 calories per kilogram or 25 to 30 calories per kilogram (depending on professional interpretation of calorie needs).

Table 1.4 Calories per kilogram estimation method for determining calorie needs

Calories per kilogram Estimation Method for Determining Calorie Needs	
To lose weight	20–25 calories per kg body weight
To maintain weight	25–30 calories per kg body weight
To gain weight	30–35 calories per kg body weight

Table 1.5 Adjusted body weight equation for use in individuals >125% ideal body weight

Determining Adjusted Body Weight (ABW) for use in Individuals >125%
ABW: [(actual body weight – ideal body weight) × 0.25] + ideal body weight

Dietary Reference Intakes

In the United States, the Food and Nutrition Board of the Institute of Medicine has developed and periodically revises the Dietary Reference Intakes (DRIs). The DRIs contain a variety of energy (calorie) and nutrient intake standards for Americans. While the DRIs encompass a number of terms and standards, the most familiar DRI is the Recommended Dietary Allowance (RDA). RDA is an amount of a nutrient that meets the nutrient needs of 98 percent of individuals in a given age and gender group. In the event that there is not enough scientific data to set the RDA for a particular nutrient, the DRI committee establishes an Adequate Intake (AI) level for that nutrient. In addition to the RDAs and AIs, nutrition scientists have also established Tolerable Upper Intake Levels (ULs), also called upper levels, for some nutrients. The UL is the highest average amount of a nutrient for a given age and gender group that is unlikely to be harmful or pose a toxicity threat when consumed daily. Not all nutrients have ULs defined, but for those that have ULs, consumers are advised not to consume that nutrient in levels above the UL. Practitioners should be aware of the DRIs in order to make nutrient and energy intake recommendations for patients of different age and gender groups, and to advise patients about potential safety concerns of supplements consumed in very high doses. The DRI Tables with recommended intakes for individuals are available online at http://www.nal.usda.gov/fnic/DRI/DRI_Tables/recommended_intakes_in dividuals.pdf.

Estimating Macronutrient Needs

Once a baseline level of calories needed per day has been established, it is helpful for the practitioner to be able to advise a client or patient on how to distribute those calories among carbohydrate, fat, and protein intake. The acceptable macronutrient distribution range (AMDR) is a DRI that provides details on how distribution of total calories should look in a well-balanced diet. AMDRs set an upper and lower range for percent of calories from the three essential macronutrients— carbohydrate, fat, and protein. Practitioners can use the AMDR to recommend grams of carbohydrate, fat, and protein for individuals' diets.

Grams of carbohydrate, fat, and protein are often more useful for consumers than calories from carbohydrate, fat, and protein as listed on the Nutrition Facts Panel. The AMDR can then be compared against current dietary intakes of patients and clients or to make recommendations about how much of each macronutrient to consume.

The AMDRs, and the scientific data from which they are derived, state that the majority of calories in a well-balanced diet should come from carbohydrate (45 to 65 percent of calories in an adult diet), with less calories coming from fat and protein (20 to 35 percent and 10 to 35 percent respectively). The AMDRs are outlined in Table 1.6 and require the practitioner to know the energy density of each macronutrient: 1 gram of carbohydrate contains 4 calories, 1 gram of fat contains 9 calories, and 1 gram of protein contains 4 calories.

No significant data exists to set forth a DRI for fat. In addition to the AMDR for fat of 20 to 35 percent of calories, practitioners may find the American Heart Association's (AHA) recommendations useful. AHA recommends that healthy Americans over age 2 eat between 25 to 35 percent of total daily calories as fats from foods like fish, nuts, and vegetable oils (AHA, 2015). The Daily Value on the food label recommends eating no more than 65 grams of fat per day when following a 2,000-calorie diet (representing 29 percent of total calories from fat). For protein, the dietary reference intake for healthy adults is 0.8 grams per kilogram body weight; however, certain medical conditions require an increase or decrease in protein compared to this level. Table 1.7 further outlines the DRIs for water, carbohydrate, fiber, and protein for different age and gender groups.

Table 1.6 AMDR for macronutrients (National Research Council, 2005)

	Macronutrient Distribution Range (percent of energy/calories)		
Macronutrient	Children, 1–3 years	Children, 4–18 years	Adults >18 years
Carbohydrate	45–65%	45–65%	45–65%
Fat	30–40%	25–35%	20–35%
Protein	5–20%	10–30%	10–35%

Table 1.7 DRIs for water, carbohydrate, dietary fiber, fat, and protein

	Total Water (L/d)[a]	Carbohydrate (g/d)	Total Fiber (g/d)	Fat (g/d)	Protein (g/d)[b]
Infants					
0–6 mo	0.7*	60*	ND[c]	31*	9.1*
6–12 mo	0.8*	95*	ND	30*	11.0
Children					
1–3 y	1.3*	130	19*	ND	13
4–8 y	1.7*	130	25*	ND	19
Males					
9–13 y	2.4*	130	31*	ND	34
14–18 y	3.3*	130	38*	ND	52
19–30 y	3.7*	130	38*	ND	56
31–50 y	3.7*	130	38*	ND	56
51–70 y	3.7*	130	30*	ND	56
>70 y	3.7*	130	30*	ND	56
Females					
9–13 y	2.1*	130	26*	ND	34
14–18 y	2.3*	130	26*	ND	46
19–30 y	2.7*	130	25*	ND	46
31–50 y	2.7*	130	25*	ND	46
51–70 y	2.7*	130	21*	ND	46
>70 y	2.7*	130	21*	ND	46
Pregnancy					
14–18 y	3.0*	175	28*	ND	71
19–30 y	3.0*	175	28*	ND	71
31–50 y	3.0*	175	28*	ND	71
Lactation					
14–18 y	3.8*	210	29*	ND	71
19–30 y	3.8*	210	29*	ND	71
31–50 y	3.8*	210	29*	ND	71

* Values marked by asterisk (*) indicate Adequate Intake (AI) values; an AI is set when there is not enough data to determine a Recommended Dietary Allowance (RDA) value. The RDA is

Total Water (L/d)[a]	Carbohydrate (g/d)	Total Fiber (g/d)	Fat (g/d)	Protein (g/d)[b]
the average daily dietary intake level sufficient to meet the nutrient requirements of nearly all (97 to 98 percent) of healthy individuals in a group. The AI is believed to cover the needs of all healthy individuals in the group, but lack of data or uncertainty in the data prevent being able to specify with confidence the percentage of individuals covered by this intake.				

a: Total water includes all water contained in food, beverages, and drinking water
b: Based on grams of protein per kg of body weight for the reference body weight; e.g., for adults 0.8 g/kg body weight for the reference body weight
c: ND: Not Determined

Estimating Micronutrient Needs

As with the macronutrients, the amount of micronutrients (vitamins and minerals) required by individuals varies by age and gender group. The full DRIs for vitamins and minerals (elements) can be found at http://www.nal.usda.gov/fnic/DRI/DRI_Tables/recommended_intakes_individuals.pdf. The DRI tables also include the tolerable ULs. While people should aim to meet the DRIs for each vitamin and mineral, they should avoid exceeding the UL as it presents an increased risk for vitamin and mineral toxicity. Individuals rarely can achieve greater-than-UL intakes of vitamins and minerals through food consumption, but using high doses of dietary supplements can easily lead a person to surpass the UL.

Interactive DRI for Health care Professionals

Interactive DRI for Health care Professionals is a web-based tool used to calculate daily nutrient recommendations for dietary planning. The tool is based on the DRIs developed by the National Academy of Science's Institute on Medicine. The practitioner enters the client's gender, age, height, weight, and activity level and then generates a detailed report of individual calorie and nutrient needs based on the DRI for that age/gender group. Useful applications of this tool include establishing minimum daily carbohydrate needs for people with diabetes, explaining baseline dietary fiber recommendations, comparing current versus recommended calcium intake, or explaining how increased physical activity affects individual energy needs. You can access the interactive DRI tool at: http://fnic.nal.usda.gov/fnic/interactiveDRI/.

Nutrition Counseling Tips and Techniques

In the profession of nutrition, utilization of information and the tactful imparting of knowledge is key to promoting behavior change. Nutrition professionals employ nutrition counseling as a means to improve overall health behaviors through the collaborative implementation of nutrition interventions. Nutrition counseling is defined as "a supportive process to set priorities, establish goals, and create individualized action plans that acknowledge and foster responsibility for self-care" (AND, 2007a). Maintaining objectivity and supporting behavior change are essential tools for nutrition counseling success. There are a number of personal characteristics and theoretical approaches that can facilitate positive behavior changes in those clients and patients who are actively engaged in nutrition counseling.

Characteristics of Effective Counseling

The goal of all nutrition educators and practitioners is to be an effective counselor. So what exactly are the characteristics of an effective counselor? There is no one prescribed answer for this complex question. Your individual approach to providing nutrition information will be much like that of your general patient interactions—highly personalized and individualized. You may be able to have a light-hearted, off-the-cuff conversation about sodium and potassium intake with one patient who has hypertension, while another may require a more calculated and directed message delivered in a serious and respectful tone. There is no "one-size-fits-all" approach when it comes to nutrition counseling. The directions you can take a patient with regards to your methods of imparting nutrition knowledge are truly limitless. While this may at first seem overwhelming, it may be helpful to note that while there is no one right way to provide nutrition counseling, it also means that there is really no one wrong way to do the same! In one study that looked at personal characteristics of effective counselors, 10 expert counselors were questioned about 22 personality characteristics that could be attributable to effective counselors. The experts ranked empathy, acceptance, and warmth as the most important characteristics, while the least important traits included resourcefulness, sympathy, and sociability (Pope & Kline, 1999).

Empathy

To express empathy means that you are identifying with and understanding the other person's feelings, beliefs, and point of view. Essentially, expressing empathy is not just about putting you in another person's shoes, but also forcing you to shift perspective (Murphy & Dillon, 1998). Take the example of organic foods. While you might personally extol the environmental and ethical reasons behind increasing organic food intake, if your client is on a minimal, fixed income and cites financial reasons behind his or her limited fruit and vegetable intake, are you being empathetic when you tout organics? Most likely not! In this situation, the empathetic thing would be to first ask, "If I were this client, why would I not be eating more fruits and vegetables?" If the answer is, "Because I don't think I can afford them," then a recommendation to buy the most expensive tier of fruits and vegetables would be inappropriate. An empathetic counselor listens patiently, processes the information internally, and seeks to truly understand the other person's perspective before responding.

To become empathetic, one must first be a good listener. Listen to your client and process what he or she is saying. Too often we become so excited to share what we know about the benefits of this and the drawbacks of that that we end up imparting information before truly understanding the issue at hand. Lastly, when considering empathy, Murphy and Dillon caution interviewers not to confuse empathy with sympathy, saying, "Empathy is not sympathy. Sympathy is what I feel toward you; empathy is what I feel as you" (Murphy & Dillon, 1998).

Supportiveness

While it is often unlikely that you can fix someone else's problems, letting that person know that you are there to support him or her can help the individual work towards solutions of their own. One way you can offer support is to provide information about what others in a similar situation have done. Consider referring individuals interested in weight loss to the National Weight Control Registry (NWCR). The NWCR was established in 1994 by researchers from Brown Medical School and the University of Colorado. It is the largest prospective investigation of long-term successful weight loss maintenance. The key to NWCR is that it tracks maintenance. Any overweight person can likely employ any number of unhealthy approaches to lose weight initially; it is more interesting, and relevant, instead, to study what healthful practices have allowed those who have had successful weight loss to *keep it off* for significant periods of time. NWCR tracks people who have lost 30 pounds and kept that weight off for at least one year or more.

Researchers then analyze what the more than 10,000 people enrolled in the registry have in common and how their exercise and eating patterns influence or have influenced their successful weight loss. Motivated clients may find inspiration and strength in the researchers' findings. For example, members in the registry have lost an average of 66 pounds and have kept it off for 5.5 years; 78 percent of the successful losers eat breakfast every day and 90 percent exercise on average at least one hour per day (National Weight Control Registry, 2012). You can learn more about the NWCR at http://www.nwcr.ws/.

Warmth

The renowned Dallas Cowboys football coach Jimmy Johnson once said, "The only thing worse than a coach or CEO who doesn't care about his people is one who pretends to care. People can spot a phony every time." Your clients and patients know exactly when you don't care; but they also know and respond positively when you *do* care. When you sit down to talk about food, nutrition, or weight—or any sensitive topic for that matter—don't be a phony. Leave your attitude, judgments, and preconceived notions at the door. Think about where people are coming from and learn where they are going.

Take the case of an overweight client named Rose. Rose is 250 pounds, and she has type 2 diabetes. If you were to meet Rose in your clinic waiting room, you might think, "Wow, Rose is huge, and I bet her blood sugar is out of control." But what you may not know is that just a year ago, Rose weighed over 350 pounds, and she had been hospitalized multiple times for diabetic ketoacidosis. A perceptive intern in the emergency department recognized Rose as having been admitted multiple times for the same diagnosis. Upon discharge the intern initiated a casual discussion with Rose about an outpatient diabetes clinic that she might consider to help her lose weight, improve her glycemic control, and ultimately eliminate the need for her to endure the recurrent, expensive, and stressful hospital admissions. The intern stressed that he was concerned for Rose's wellbeing and recommended the clinic as a means to help her out. Rose reacted positively to the intern's warmth and concern for her well-being, and she eventually enrolled in the diabetes self-management program. She has been working with the clinic's diabetes educators on gradually losing weight, improving her diet, and increasing her exercise capacity. Rose is not at her goal, but she is getting there, and all it took was the warmth of a concerned health care practitioner to redirect her path from a downward health spiral to a more healthful direction. Now that you know Rose's story, do you see her in a different light as she sits in your waiting room?

When you are prepared to broach the topic of nutrition or food with your patients, be yourself. Have a strategy, but be conversational and try to avoid overly technical language or medical jargon. Talk in frank terms about evidence-based strategies for improving health with nutrition. And above all, always keep in mind that you cannot judge a book by the cover: you must take the time to read the whole story.

Theoretical Approaches to Nutrition Counseling

There are a number of theoretical approaches to nutrition counseling that can be enacted to affect behavior change. In the one-on-one or group counseling environment, it may be helpful to think of yourself more as a coach than as a teacher. If you keep goal-setting a person-centered and patient-directed activity, you can help guide your clients to set, plan for, work towards, and achieve their own goals. Ultimately, however, *they* need to be in the driver's seat if the changes are truly going to "stick" and work.

The Health Belief Model

The Health Belief Model (HBM) was developed in the 1950s to help social psychologists in the U.S. Public Health Service more clearly understand why people did not participate in programs designed to prevent and detect disease (Hochbaum, 1958), (Rosenstock, 1960). HBM is constructed on the assumptions that a negative health condition or disease state is avoidable, that taking a particular action can lead to avoidance of such a condition or disease state, and that the individual maintains the power to exert control over the behavior that can lead to positive changes or outcomes.

For example, an individual with chronic kidney disease can choose to acknowledge that chronic kidney disease is not inevitable, that limiting phosphorus intake can mitigate kidney damage, and that with the right amount of knowledge and education, the person can control his phosphorus intake in order to improve kidney function. Table 1.8 outlines the basic constructs of the HBM.

Table 1.8 *Health belief model constructs and nutrition application*

Health Belief Model Construct	Definition	Nutrition Application Perception Statement
Perceived susceptibility	Belief about the likelihood of contracting a disease or getting a particular medical condition	"I believe that because my family has a strong history of colon cancer that I also am at risk for colon cancer."
Perceived severity	Belief about how serious a disease or medical condition is	"My uncle had diabetes and lost his left foot. I know it is a serious condition with life-changing consequences."
Perceived benefits	Belief in the effectiveness of recommended actions to reduce risk or severity of disease or medical condition	"If I work on decreasing my saturated fat and increasing my dietary fiber, maybe I can avoid having to take a statin drug for my cholesterol."
Perceived barriers	Belief about impediments to success in preventing or treating the disease or medical condition	"Only rich people can afford all the fruits and vegetables I should probably be eating to help me lose weight."

Health Belief Model Construct	Definition	Nutrition Application Perception Statement
Cues to action	Strategies intended to promote readiness	"When I learned that I had prediabetes and that it meant I might get diabetes, I got scared and decided to do something about by eating habits."
Self-efficacy	Belief or confidence in one's own ability to take positive action	"I know it's going to be hard to maintain a gluten-free diet to help my celiac disease, but I saw my neighbor do it, and I think I can do it too."

The Transtheoretical Model and Stages of Change

The Transtheoretical Model, also called the Stages of Change Model, is applicable in many counseling environments and can also be helpful in identifying where a client is at with regards to his or her readiness to change nutrition behaviors. The model has been designed to help explain behavior changes related to smoking cessation, stress management, and diet improvements, and it consists of six stages: precontemplation, contemplation, preparation, action, maintenance, and termination. In some models, relapse is added as a seventh stage. The practitioner can use the Stages of Change to determine what stage a particular learner or patient may be at. Table 1.9 defines the individual stages and provides an application statement for each stage based on an individual who has received a recommendation to begin walking 30 minutes per day in order to control high blood pressure as an alternative to beginning on a blood pressure lowering medication.

Table 1.9 Stages of change and nutrition application (Glanz, Rimer, & Viswanath, 2008), (AND, 2015h)

Stage	Definition	Sample Statement at Stage	Techniques for Counselor
Precontemplation	No intention to take any action within the next 6 months	"I'm really busy at work right now and probably will be through the holidays and then into tax season. Starting a walking	• Validate lack of readiness. • Help clients to clarify that the decision belongs

Stage	Definition	Sample Statement at Stage	Techniques for Counselor
		program right now just isn't going to work with my schedule."	to them. • Encourage reevaluation of current behaviors. • Encourage self-exploration (not action).
Contemplation	Intends to take action within the next 6 months	"OK, I am too young to be so out of breath just walking up these stairs! I think by my birthday I need to get into a routine where I walk every day to get in shape."	• Validate lack of readiness. • Help clients to clarify that the decision belongs to them. • Encourage evaluation of pros and cons of behavior change. • Identify and promote new, positive outcome expectations.
Preparation	Intends to take action within the next 30 days and has taken some behavioral steps in this direction	"Those new walking shoes I just bought were sure expensive. But it is an investment in my health, and I am going to use them soon, no matter what!"	• Identify and assist in problem solving. • Assist client to identify social supports. • Verify that client has the underlying skills for behavior change. • Encourage initial small steps.
Action	Changed overt behavior for less than 6 months	"I've been walking on my lunch break every day for a few weeks now, and I'm surprised it wasn't as bad as I thought it would be."	• Continue reinforcing the decision to act. • Focus on restructuring cues and social support.

Stage	Definition	Sample Statement at Stage	Techniques for Counselor
			• Promote self-efficacy for handling obstacles. • Combat feelings of loss by echoing long-term benefits that the client has identified.
Maintenance	Changed overt behavior for more than 6 months	"I've been walking either on my lunch break or before or after work for 30 minutes every weekday, for the last 9 months."	• Plan for follow-up support. • Reinforce internal rewards and health benefits. • Discuss coping with relapse.
Termination, or in alternate case, Relapse	Termination: No temptation to relapse and 100% confidence Relapse: Resumption of previous behavior	"Doing my daily walk is now just part of my routine. I don't even think twice about it. I know that it helps keep my weight at a good spot and my blood pressure down, and most importantly, I don't have to take any medications." Relapse statement (patient reverts to Preparation phase): "I have stopped walking and am back to my old sedentary ways. But I'll bring my shoes with me to work tomorrow so I can exercise in my lunch break."	• For relapse: evaluate triggers for relapse—what caused the relapse? • Reassess motivation and barriers.

Cognitive Behavioral Therapy

Cognitive Behavioral Therapy (CBT) represents the blending of two therapies, cognitive therapy (CT) and behavioral therapy (National Institute of Mental Health, 2015). CBT assumes that behaviors are learned and that these behaviors are linked to both internal and external triggers that lead to problem behavior. CBT encourages the person to examine his or her thoughts and beliefs, to analyze how they affect moods and actions, and to direct changes in behavior that reflect a more positive health outlook. With CBT, the intervention targets identification of erroneous thoughts and beliefs, such as, "I can't lose weight" or "carbohydrates are fattening," and modifies those thoughts and beliefs. With behavioral therapy, individuals are encouraged to experience a heightened awareness of environmental triggers to eating (smells, emotions, social situations, etc.) and to modify those stimuli and responses (AND, 2015g). Practitioners of CBT may encourage participants to keep records and journals of eating events, associated feelings and emotions, surroundings, and other thoughts and beliefs in order to identify triggers of problematic behavior. Other cognitive behavior strategies include goal setting, action planning, management of barriers, and self-monitoring (Gohner, Schlatterer, Seelig, Frey, Berg, & Fuchs, 2012).

Motivational Interviewing

Although motivational interviewing (MI) was originally developed to address addictive behavior, it is also adaptable for use in nutrition counseling. MI assumes that people digress from their path to goal achievement due to a lack of motivation. Motivational interviewing has been described as "an empathetic person-centered counseling approach that prepares people for change by helping them resolve ambivalence, enhance intrinsic motivation, and build confidence to change" (Kraybill & Morrison, 2007). One way in which the motivational interview can promulgate change is by practicing OARS: asking Open-ended questions, providing Affirmation statements, practicing Reflective listening and Summarizing (Miller & Rollnick, 2002). The motivational interviewer works to promote a focus on strategies that will help motivate the client to build the commitment required to make a behavior change (Bauer & Sokolik, 2002). The basic principles of MI are outlined in Table 1.10 and specific strategies involved in MI are covered in Table 1.11.

*Table 1.10 Basic principles of motivational interviewing (Bauer &
Sokolik, 2002)*

Basic Principles of Motivational Interviewing
Express Empathy
Put yourself in the other person's shoes in order to understand that person's perspective.
Develop Discrepancy
Highlight and intensify obvious discrepancies between current behavior and stated goals to the point where changing from current behavior becomes the recognizable course of action.
Avoid Escalating Resistance
Monitor for and avoid approaching signs of resistance, such as discussions that become argumentative, reluctant or full of denial; change course if resistance escalates.
Roll with Resistance
When resistance does occur, go with it; create a supportive environment where the client can contemplate expressing fears about change without feeling judged.
Support Self-Efficacy
Promote the client's belief and confidence that he or she can achieve the stated goal.

*Table 1.11 Strategies for motivational interviewing (Rollnick,
Heather, & Bell, 1992)*

Strategies for Motivational Interviewing
Allow clients to come to their own conclusions about pros and cons of the proposed change.
Assist with, but do not push clients into making decisions.
Give examples of how others in similar situations have acted or decided.
Reinforce the idea that ultimately, the client is the best judge of what will work.
Do not project your ideas about how the client should feel regarding his or her condition.
Present an array of options and choices.
Clarify goals when necessary.
Acknowledge that failing to reach a decision to change does not constitute a failed session.
Anticipate fluctuating levels of commitment.
Express empathy with the client's situation.

Table 1.12 The OARS of motivational interviewing (Miller &
Rollnick, 2002)

The OARS of Motivational Interviewing
Open-Ended Questioning
Affirmations
Reflective Listening
Summaries

Nutrition Counseling Tips for Individuals

Your individual nutrition counseling style is more likely to be a compilation of bits and pieces of the aforementioned models and constructs than to one that fits nicely into one of the defined boxes. Just as there is no one diet or weight-loss plan that works for all people, there is no one approach to nutrition counseling that is appropriate for all patient types. The following recommendations are provided for you to consider as you work towards becoming more comfortable broaching sensitive food and diet topics with your patients and to help you develop your own nutrition counseling style.

Use Evidence-Based Medicine

Take a look around our food environment, and you will see that opinions are everywhere—*this* is the new super food, *that* is the new quick-fix diet. It seems that everywhere we are being pushed in different directions with regards to food and nutrition. One day butter is better for you, the next day margarine is. Egg yolks are in; egg yolks are out. Eat small frequent meals; never eat between meals. How can a busy practitioner possibly process and stay on top of all of this information, not to mention put it into usable form for the patients and clients?

If you start to feel overwhelmed about your ability to stay on top of the latest food and nutrition information, save your sanity by turning to evidence-based medicine. The term evidence-based medicine (EBM) is thought to have first been used by investigators from McMaster University during the 1990s. EBM has been defined as "a systemic approach to analyze published research as the basis of clinical decision making", and then more formally defined by Sacket et al., who stated that EBM was "the conscientious and judicious use of current best evidence from clinical care research in the management of individual patients" (Claridge & Fabian, 2005). In our lightning-fast era of web searches, quasi-professionals, and self-diagnoses, the validity of EBM far surpasses any other sources of information. On the other hand, not using EBM may challenge your professional liability.

In our rapidly evolving health care and food environments, we are constantly inundated with information. Patients and clients turn to practitioners to help them decipher confusing and conflicting messages. It is certainly a challenge to stay current, but there are an ever-increasing number of resources to help you do so. While you can never read all of the most recent published scientific literature, there are credible newsletters that will summarize it for you. Consider subscribing to mailed, hard copy summary health letters such as University of California, Berkeley's *Wellness Letter*, The Center for Science in the Public Interest's (CSPI) *Nutrition Action Health Letter*, and *Tufts Health and Nutrition Letter Sign*. Get electronic news and updates from reputable nutrition sources such as the Harvard School of Public Health's The Nutrition Source page, Nutrition.gov, or the Mayo Clinic, and sign up for your professional association's weekly email newsletters.

Another way to stay current is to be aware of what is obsolete. In nutrition, diet therapies that have been shown to be ineffective through scientific research have a habit of sticking around in day-to-day practice long after they have been disproven. For example, in the past, geriatric patients would be placed on overly restricted diets (e.g., low-cholesterol, low-fat, sodium-restricted, calorie-controlled diabetic diets) while in hospitals or long-term care facilities; however, authoritative nutrition bodies now assert that these overly restrictive diet orders should be avoided because they promote inadequate nutrient intake in these individuals (AND, 2015g). The overarching goal of nutrition therapy for those who are ill is to promote the least-restrictive diet. Promoting liberalized diets may involve a certain level of "unlearning" on the part of the practitioner, who hears, sees, and reads about specific dietary recommendations for disease states but does not understand that ordering such a restrictive diet may actually promote undernutrition in sick patients.

Table 1.13 Tips for establishing rapport in a counseling session

Tips for Establishing Rapport in a Counseling Session
Do your background research before the client arrives, and greet the client by name.
Use a firm but not overpowering handshake and make eye contact when greeting the client.
Introduce yourself briefly and then ask open-ended questions to the client for his or her introduction.
Avoid the urge to interrupt unnecessarily, to pass judgment, or to convey bias in your communications.
Offering the client a glass of water, coffee, or tea may help set the stage for a conversational rather than confrontational session.

Establish Rapport

As with any new relationship, establishing good rapport is an essential first step in the nutrition counseling process. Rapport can be defined as a harmonious relation. Without this good foundation of rapport, your counseling session can quickly go awry. Human beings are naturally reticent to talk about highly personal and sensitive topics such as weight, exercise, diet, and disease. If you make your patients feel comfortable with you and create a judgment-free zone and environment, they are going to be more likely to divulge information that will be essential for patient-driven problem solving. Table 1.13 contains some tips for establishing rapport in a counseling session.

Acknowledge Different Learning Styles

An effective counselor acknowledges that there are many different types of learners. When it comes to food and nutrition, your experience with learning styles is likely to run the gamut. You will encounter the type who says, "Just tell me what to eat and I'll do it!", while your next patient may say, "If you teach me about carbohydrates, I can work them into my meal planning for diabetes management." Some people are more number oriented and want percentages and numbers of calories, while others are word oriented and respond well to "eat more" and "eat less" messages. There are visual learners who will easily conceptualize portion size comparisons when given standard household measurements, but there are also kinesthetic learners who will conceptualize portion sizes by touching and feeling food models. Be prepared to counsel using various techniques because not everyone learns in the same manner. A few simple questions directed at the outset of your session or appointment regarding the patient's preferred learning style can help set you, as the educator, on the right path.

Individualize Your Approach

Just as a prescribed calorie level for all people with diabetes has fallen out of favor, so has the one-size-fits-all approach to nutrition counseling. The conventional wisdom now maintains that any nutrition information you disseminate should be individualized and tailored to fit the patient or client. Whereas *you* may eat three meals per day, your client might work a swing shift schedule that impedes his or her ability to do so. A plan that works for one person might not be appropriate for another. Ask clients to tell you about their usual day, their typical eating patterns, personal diet and weight history, and perceived barriers to success in order to provide you with data needed to create an individualized meal plan. Chapter 1 contains more information on healthy meal planning.

Avoid Bias

The term social distance refers to the variations in characteristics that may exist in the clinician-patient relationship (Glanz, Rimer, & Viswanath, 2008). Age, race, gender, and lifestyle have the potential to either strengthen or lessen the patient-provider bond. In a judgment-free environment, practitioners are encouraged to express empathy, share understanding, show attentiveness, and ask questions about the patients' beliefs and value system in order to elicit communication, respect, and information from the client that can help improve his or her nutritional status.

Practice Reflective Listening

- Reflective listening is an essential skill for an effective listener to have. It helps fill in gaps in communication and to avoid misunderstanding. There are three primary levels of reflective listening (Substance Abuse and Mental Health Services Administration's (SAMHSA) Homelessness Resource Center (HRC), 2007):
- Repeating or rephrasing: listener uses synonyms or substitutes phrases, staying close to what the speaker has said
- Paraphrasing: listener provides a restatement that reaffirms the tone and intent of what speaker has said
- Reflection of feeling: listener highlights the emotional content of speakers' statements—this is considered to be the deepest form of listening Examples of reflective listening statements include, "So you feel like cutting back on your number of fast food meals is going to be a challenge?", "It sounds like you have identified a number of higher-fiber fruit options that you can take to work for between meal snacks," and "You are wondering if reducing the amount of wine you drink is going to affect your ability to have a good time in social situations." While restating the patient's words may seem repetitive, it ensures that you understand what they are saying, and it gives them the opportunity to clarify information that may have previously been misinterpreted.

Ask Open-Ended Questions

Open-ended questions allow respondents to tell their own story without feeling that they have to take the answer in a prescribed direction. One way to think about asking more open-ended questions is to focus on asking *less* closed questions. A closed question is one that leads the respondent in a particular direction—more simply put, a yes/no question. "Did you have breakfast this morning?" implies that I, as the counselor expect that you, as the respondent, eat breakfast. Even if you didn't eat breakfast, you might *say* you did because the question indicates that the questioner places some value on this thing called "breakfast." Additionally, including "this morning" as a part of the question implies that I think you woke up in the morning, which, depending upon your schedule or personal preference, could be entirely untrue. A better way to reframe that question as an open-ended question would be to ask, "Tell me about the first thing or things you ate or drank after getting up today". More examples of open question lead-ins include:

- How can I help you with _____?
- Help me understand _____?
- When are you most likely to _____?
- When have you tried before to make a change?
- When might you be most ready to _____?
- How would you like things to be different?
- What are the good things about _____ and what are the less-than-good things about _____? (Substance Abuse and Mental Health Services Administration's (SAMHSA) Homelessness Resource Center (HRC, 2007)

When asking open-ended questions, start with words like who, what, when, where, how, and why as opposed to words like did, could, and would.

Set SMART Goals

The Academy of Nutrition and Dietetics recommends the following sequence of steps for helping clients set goals related to diet. The practitioner needs to do the following:

- Facilitate client identification of nutrition-related goals
- Evaluate the pros and cons of goal(s) and asks the client to prioritize one goal
- Ask the client to describe how he or she plans to accomplish the goal and ask questions to help the client clarify important details of the plan

- Determine when, where, and how frequently they will do this
- Identify a way to measure if the goal was attained
- Identify nutrition subgoals (e.g., a subgoal for a long-term goal of eliminating less than healthful snacks would be to eliminate the morning doughnut snack and determine a realistic alternative)
- Establish client commitment, including the identification of obstacles that might prevent goal attainment and providing resources that may be helpful in goal achievement

When working with clients to craft goals and objectives, aim for outcomes that adhere to the SMART criteria. A SMART objective is one that is specific, measurable, achievable, realistic, and time-phased or timely. Table 1.14 contains more detail on writing SMART objectives.

Table 1.14 Writing SMART goals and objectives (CDC, 2009)

Writing SMART Goals and Objectives	
Specific	• Limit to one action verb • Avoid vague terms • The more specific, the more measurable the outcome is
Measurable	• Focus on "how much" change is desired • Objective should provide a reference point from which deviation and change can be measured
Achievable	• Attainable within a time frame • Attainable with given resources
Realistic	• Accurately address the scope of the problem • If objective does not directly relate to the goal, it is not helpful
Time-phased	• Time frame indicating when objective will be accomplished • Time-phased goals set the stage for planning and evaluation of the intervention

Assign Homework

Although you may think of homework in the context of younger patients and clients, you may be surprised to learn that many adults actually *like* homework! As a part of your goal setting in nutrition counseling, consider assigning homework to your client to complete between sessions. As a part of your summary statements at the end of a session, you might work with the client to identify, for example, two food-related and one exercise-related homework assignments. Keep these assignments client-directed, remembering that you "telling" someone what to do in the next day/week/month is less effective than that person telling you what he or is she is likely to do. Examples of food-related homework may include:

- I will take two pieces of fruit with me to work for my between-meal snacks; I will place them on my desk and not let myself leave work until I have eaten those two pieces of fruit.
- I will go through my pantry and remove all the processed and packaged high-salt and high-fat junk foods and either throw them out or donate them.
- I will measure out the amount of fluid allowed by my fluid restriction at the beginning of each day for the next week to help me stay within my fluid limits.
- I will try one new vegetable before our next session.

Examples of exercise-related homework assignments:

- I will go for a 20 minute walk in my lunch break at least one day during this upcoming work week.
- I will reactivate my gym membership this week.
- I will find an exercise partner who I can work out with at least two times per week before our next session.

When working with clients on identifying useful homework assignments, start small and think baby steps. As a provider, your goal in this role might be as simple as to help your clients stay reasonable. If Barbara hasn't been off the couch in months, it is unlikely that she will immediately start going to the gym six days in a week. Even if she does, the change is too dramatic, making it is unlikely to result in sustainable behavior change. A more realistic homework assignment might be for Barbara to walk around the block five separate times before your next session.

Track Outcomes Other Than Weight

Too often in nutrition counseling, the focus is on weight. "I lost five pounds, and I feel great" can easily turn into, "I didn't lose as much weight as I wanted to this week, and now I feel discouraged." Encourage your clients to focus on positive outcomes that *don't* come from the scale. It is inspiring for patients to be able to tighten their belts one more notch, to watch their pant size go down, and for them to see muscles develop where fat once existed. Celebrate non-weight related victories such as improvements in lab values, reductions in blood pressure, increasing exercise capacity, and improved sleep patterns. For weight loss, while it is important to track weight regularly, highlight other areas of progress to discourage an overemphasis on weight. Many clients are inclined to weigh themselves every morning in order to track their weight loss, but this may set them up for disappointment. It may be prudent to have them only weigh themselves one time per week, or once every two weeks, in order to focus on the behaviors they are changing, as opposed to a number on the scale.

Plan for Pitfalls

Thomas Edison once said, "I have not failed. I've just found 10,000 ways that won't work." Your journey with patients to their food and nutrition goals will no doubt encounter obstacles, roadblocks, and failures. Relationships do not disintegrate because of setbacks, but rather because of an inability to deal with setbacks. As a practitioner, you are the coach that helps your clients and patients deal with setbacks. In anticipation of potential hiccups, be proactive and brainstorm with your clients what might go wrong with the set plan. In diet therapy, it may help to think of an informal approach called "cruise management". If a client is getting ready to go on a cruise, he or she is going to encounter a pretty predictable food situation: trapped on a boat in the middle of the ocean with innumerable opportunities to eat coupled with an inherent pressure to eat like you're getting your money's worth! Visualize scenarios that may arise, talk about how the scenario might be handled, and offer suggestions for mitigating damage. Holidays, social gatherings, and family reunions present challenging environments for keeping to a set plan. Setbacks are inevitable, but being prepared for those inevitable setbacks promotes success. Remind your clients, "If you fail to plan, you plan to fail."

Group Counseling

The group approach to nutrition counseling is not designed to be a form of therapy, but rather to create an environment that seeks to find solutions to common nutrition problems (Helm, 1995). In some cases, group counseling may provide advantages that are not attainable in the one-on-one setting, such as emotional support and group problem solving. In groups, participants have the opportunity to learn from each other through what is known as the "modeling effect". Additionally, group participants encourage each other to reevaluate their own belief systems through the interactions and experiences with others in the group. Potential drawbacks of group counseling include reticent individuals not having their opinions or voices heard, personality differences leading to one or a few members dominating the discussion, poor role modeling, and the facilitator not being able to meet the needs of all group members (Bauer & Sokolik, 2002). Table 1.15 contains a list of some helpful tips for successfully facilitating a group counseling session.

Table 1.15 Tips for leading successful group counseling sessions

Tips for Successfully Facilitating a Group Counseling Session
Set the stage: Select an appropriate room and environment with a seating arrangement that is conducive to sharing ideas; closing the door may promote a feeling of security.
Limit the size: An ideal group size is 6 to 12 people.
Build a better group: Interview prospective members, group people together with common interests or health conditions, some mix may be good but too much disparity may confuse participants.
Encourage buy-in: Collecting a fee can encourage attendance as participants have a sense of ownership; conduct financial business at the beginning of the meeting.
Be consistent: The same person should lead the group each session.
Run a tight ship: Arrive early, start and conclude at scheduled times, provide session overview, follow a lesson plan, redirect inappropriate conversation.
Be proactive about attendance: Call those who missed the meeting, inquire about reasons for not attending, and express concern for well-being to help retention.

References

Academy of Nutrition and Dietetics. 2007. *Nutrition Care Process.* Retrieved September 26, 2012 from Evidence Analysis Library: http://andevidence library.com.

Academy of Nutrition and Dietetics. 2007a. *What Is the Evidence Regarding the Difference in Effectiveness for Individual- vs. Group-based Nutrition Counseling?* Retrieved September 30, 2015, from Evidence Analysis Library: http://andevidencelibrary.com.

Academy of Nutrition and Dietetics. 2009. *ADA Conclusion Statements and Accuracy of Resting Metabolic Rate Measurement vs. Estimations.* Retrieved September 26, 2012, from Evidence Analysis Library: http://andevidencelibrary.com.

Academy of Nutrition and Dietetics. 2013. *Why Adding an RD to Your Practice Team Is Good Medicine.* Retrieved September 30, 2015, from RDs and PCPs: A Healthy Partnership for the Comprehensive Primary Care Initiative: www.eatrightpro.org/~/media/eatrightpro%20files/career/career%20development/marketing%20center/online%20marketing%20center%20documents/why%20adding%20an%20rd%20to%20your%20practice%20team%20is%20good%20medicine.ashx.

Academy of Nutrition and Dietetics. 2014. *RDNs and Medical Nutrition Therapy Services.* Retrieved September 30, 2015, from www.eatright.org/resource/food/resources/learn-more-about-rdns/rdns-and-medical-nutrition-therapy-services.

Academy of Nutrition and Dietetics. 2015. *About ACEND.* Retrieved September 29, 2015, from Accreditation Council for Eduation in Nutrition and Dietetics: www.eatrightacend.org/ACEND/.

Academy of Nutrition and Dietetics. 2015a. *About ACEND: ACEND Mission, Vision and Straregic Plan.* Retrieved September 29, 2015, from ACEND: www.eatrightacend.org/ACEND/content.aspx?id=6442485282.

Academy of Nutrition and Dietetics. 2015b. *About Us.* Retrieved September 29, 2015, from eatrightPRO: www.eatrightpro.org/resources/about-us.

Academy of Nutrition and Dietetics. 2015c. *Academy Vision and Mission.* Retrieved September 29, 2015, from About Us: www.eatrightpro.org/resources/about-us/academy-vision-and-mission.

Academy of Nutrition and Dietetics. 2015d. *Become an RDN or DTR.* Retrieved September 28, 2015, from Career: www.eatrightpro.org /resources/career/become-an-rdn-or-dtr.

Academy of Nutrition and Dietetics. 2015e. *List of Dietetic Practice Groups (DPGs).* Retrieved September 29, 2015, from eatrightPRO: www.eatrightpro.org/resource/membership/academy-groups/dietetic-practice-groups/list-of-dietetic-practice-groups.

Academy of Nutrition and Dietetics. 2015f. *List of Member Interest Groups (MIGs).* Retrieved September 29, 2015, from eatrightPRO: www.eatrightpro.org/resource/membership/academy-groups/member -interest-groups/member-interest-groups.

Academy of Nutrition and Dietetics. 2015g. *Nutrition Counseling.* Retrieved September 30, 2015, from Nutrition Care Manual: www.nutritioncaremanual.org.

Academy of Nutrition and Dietetics. 2015h. *Weight Management.* Retrieved September 30, 2015, from Nutrition Care Manual: www .nutritioncaremanual.org.

American Heart Association. 2015. *Know Your Fats.* Retrieved September 29, 2015, from Conditions: www.heart.org/HEARTORG/Conditions /Cholesterol/PreventionTreatmentofHighCholesterol/Know-Your-Fats_ UCM_305628_Article.jsp.

Bauer, K. and C. Sokolik. 2002. *Basic Nutrition Counseling Skill Development.* Belmont, CA: Wadsworth/Thomson Learning.

Centers for Disease Control and Prevention. 2008. *Establishing Rapport.* Retrieved September 22, 2012, from Behavioral Risk Factor Surveillance System: www.cdc.gov/brfss/training/interviewer /04_section/11_rapport.htm.

Centers for Disease Control and Prevention. 2009. *Program Evaluation: Healthy Youth.* Retrieved September 30, 2015, from Writing SMART Objectives: www.cdc.gov/healthyyouth/evaluation/pdf/brief3b.pdf.

Centers for Disease Control and Prevention. 2014. *Facts about Physical Activity.* Retrieved September 28, 2015, from Physical Activity: www.cdc.gov/physicalactivity/data/facts.html.

Centers for Disease Control and Prevention. 2015. *Leading Causes of Death.* Retrieved September 28, 2015, from FastStats: www.cdc.gov/nchs /fastats/leading-causes-of-death.htm.

Centers for Disease Control and Prevention. 2015a. *Obesity and Overweight.* Retrieved September 28, 2015, from FastStats: www.cdc.gov/nchs /fastats/obesity-overweight.htm.

Claridge, J. and T. Fabian. May, 2005. "History and Development of Evidence-Based Medicine." *World Journal of Surgery* 5, pp. 547–53.

Contento, I. 2011. *Nutrition Education: Linking Research, Theory, and Practice.* 2nd ed. Sudbury, MA: Jones and Bartlett.

Finkelstein, E., J. Trogdon, J. Cohen, and W. Dietz. September–October, 2009. "Annual Medical Spending Attributable to Obesity: Payer-and-Service-Specific Estimates." *Health Affairs* 28, no. 5, pp. w822–31.

Food Marketing Institute. 2014. *Shopping for Health 2014.*

Glanz, K., B. Rimer, and K. Viswanath. 2008. *Health Behavior and Health Education: Theory, Research, and Practice.* 4th ed. San Francisco, CA: Jossey-Bass.

Gohner, W., M. Schlatterer, H. Seelig, I. Frey, A. Berg, and R. Fuchs. July–August, 2012. "Two-year follow-up of an interdisciplinary cognitive-behavioral intervention program for obese adults." *The Journal of Psychology* 146, no. 4, pp. 371–91.

Helm, K. 1995. "Group Process." In *Nutrition Therapy Advanced Counseling Skills*, eds. K. Helm, and B. Klawitter. Lake Dallas, TX: Helm Seminars, pp. 207–13.

Hochbaum, G. 1958. *Public Participateion in Medical Screening Programs: A Socio-Psychological Study.* Washington, DC: US Department of Health, Education, and Welfare.

King, J.C. February, 2007. "An Evidence-Based Approach for Establishing Dietary Guidelines." *The Journal of Nutrition* 137, pp. 480–3.

Kraybill, K. and S. Morrison. 2007. *Assessing Health, Promoting Wellness: A Guide for Non-Medical Providers of Care for People Experiencing Homelessness.* Rockville, MD: Center for Mental Health Services, Substance Abuse and Mental Health Services Administration.

Lee, R.D. and D.C. Nieman. 2007. *Nutritional Assessment.* New York, NY: McGraw Hill.

Miller, W. and S. Rollnick. 2002. Motivational Interviewing Second Edition, Preparing People for Change. New York, NY: The Guilford Press.

Murphy, B. and C. Dillon. 1998. *Interviewing in Action: Process and Practice.* Pacific Grove, CA: Brooks/Cole.

National Institute of Mental Health. 2015. *Health Topics.* Retrieved September 30, 2015, from Psychotherapies: www.nimh.nih.gov/health/topics/psychotherapies/index.shtml.

National Research Council. 2005. Dietary Reference Intakes for Energy, Carbohydrate, Fiber, Fat, Fatty Acids, Cholesterol, Protein, and Amino Acids (Macronutrients). Washington, DC: The National Academies Press.

National Weight Control Registry. 2012. *NWCR Facts.* Retrieved September 30, 2015, from www.nwcr.ws/Research/default.htm.

Ogden, C., K. Flegal, M. Carroll, and C. Johnson. October, 2002. "Prevalence and trends in overweight among US children and adolescents, 1999–2000." *JAMA* 288, no. 14, pp. 1728–32.

Olshansky, S., D. Passaro, R. Hershow, J. Layden, B. Carnes, J. Brody, L. Hayflick, R.N. Butler, D.B. Allison, D.S. Ludwig. March, 2005. "A Potential Decline in Life Expectancy in the United States in the 21st Century." *The New England Journal of Medicine* 352, no. 11, pp. 1138–45.

Pope, V. and W. Kline. June, 1999. "The Personal Characteristics of Effective Counselors: What 10 Experts Think." *Psychological Reports* 84, no. 3 Pt 2, pp. 1339–44.

Rollnick, S., N. Heather, and A. Bell. 1992. "Negotiating Behavior Change in Medical Settings: The Development of Brief Motivational Interviewing." *Journal of Mental Health* 1, pp. 25–37.

Rosenstock, I. March, 1960. "What Research in Motivation Suggests for Public Health." *American Journal of Public Health and the Nations Health* 50, pp. 295–302.

Society for Nutrition Education and Behavior. 2014. *Guiding Principles and Values of SNEB & SNEB Foundation.* Retrieved September 30, 2015, from www.sneb.org/about/mission.html.

Substance Abuse and Mental Health Services Administration's (SAMHSA) Homelessness Resource Center (HRC). 2007. *Homelessness Resource Center Library.* Retrieved September 30, 2015, from Motivational Interviewing: Open Questions, Affirmation, Reflective Listening, and Summary Reflections (OARS): http://homeless.samhsa.gov/Resource/View.aspx?id=32840&AspxAutoDetectCookieSupport=1.

Troiano, R., D. Berrigan, K. Dodd, L. Masse, T. Tilert, and M. McDowell. January, 2008. "Physical Activity in the United States Measured by Accelerometer." *Medicine and Science in Sports and Exercise* 40, pp. 181–8.

Trust for America's Health and the Robert Wood Johnson Foundation. 2015. *The State of Obesity: Better Policies for a Healthier America.*

US Department of Agriculture. 2010. *USDA's Nutrition Evidence Library (NEL).* Retrieved September 22, 2012, from www.nutrition evidencelibrary.gov/.

US Department of Agriculture, Economic Research Service. 2014. *Food Consumption and Nutrient Intakes.* Retrieved September 28, 2015, from Data Products: www.ers.usda.gov/Data/FoodConsumption.

US Department of Health and Human Services. 2001. *The Surgeon General's Call to Action to Prevent and Decrease Overweight and Obesity 2001.* Rockville: US Department of Health and Human Services, Public Health Service, Office of the Surgeon General.

US Department of Health and Human Services. 2008. *Physical Activity Guidelines for Americans.* Washington, DC: US Government Printing Office.

Wolf, A., J. Crowther, J. Nadler, and V. Bovbjerg. 2009. The return on investment of a lifestyle intervention: The ICAN Program. *Accepted for presentation at the American Diabetes Association 69th Scientific Sessions (169-OR).* New Orleans.

CHAPTER 2

The History of Dietetics in North America

Chapter Abstract

Today the term dietitian conjures up images of a credentialed nutrition professional working to help individuals, groups, and institutions utilize food to maximize health outcomes. But the profession of nutrition and dietetics has come a long way since the American Dietetic Association was founded in 1917. This chapter seeks to outline a brief history of dietetic practice in North America, largely following the establishment and progression of the Academy of Nutrition and Dietetics (AND), formerly known as the American Dietetic Association (ADA).

Historical Practice of Dietetics

It is safe to say that for as long as people have been eating food, dietetics has been practiced in some form or another. The name of the field dietetics is derived from *dieto*, meaning diet or food. Over time, as society advances, the interest in studying the impact of our intake on health has shifted from trying to obtain enough food to sustain life to trying to avoid excess consumption. Whereas populations were once more likely to suffer from inadequate intake, we now are faced with many developed and developing nations which experience the opposite of the problem: access to too much food—and the wrong types of food—that negatively impact health.

As far back as biblical times, there is documentation regarding recommendations about food selection. Doctors such as Hippocrates and others developed theories about the interplay between food and an individual's health condition (ADA, 1985). It was not until the end of the

19th century and early part of the 20th century that the study of nutrition really took off with the identification and discovery of nutrients. Prior to this point, revelations about food and its impact on our body had been speculative at best.

In 1747 James Lind conducted a study testing six different treatments for 12 sailors inflicted with scurvy. He found that only lemons and limes were successful in treating the condition, and in 1753 Lind published *Treatise of Scurvy* outlining his discovery that these fruits helped to prevent scurvy in sailors who were out at sea for extended periods of time. It was later discovered that the chemical compound vitamin C was responsible for scurvy prevention, and this was eventually given the name ascorbic acid. The naming of the new vitamin was essentially paying homage to what had previously only been called the "antiscorbutic" or "anti-scurvy" factor prior to its discovery (Beeuwkes 1948). Today we take it for granted that vitamin C helps prevent scurvy, but it is estimated that over two million sailors suffered and died from the disease prior to the understanding of the relationship between diet and this particular deficiency disease (Carpenter 2012).

America's First Dietitian

Sara Tyson Heston Rorer (1849–1937) is credited with being the first dietitian in the United States. Her reputation for teaching doctors, nurses, and medical students about proper dietary practices, especially for the sick, earned her the reputation as "America's first dietitian" (Sholly 2013). Rorer was attracted to cooking and nutrition as a child, when she took an interest in her pharmacist father's work. She spent her adult years in Philadelphia and was respected by the medical community there, often being asked to speak about food and health during her frequent lectures at the medical school. She was eventually asked to develop a diet kitchen in Philadelphia where the physicians could refer patients with complex problems and order therapeutic variations of traditional foods (Rorer 1934). Rorer spoke at the World's Fair in 1893 and is the source of notable quotes about diet and health, including, "A man may eat until he can eat no more and still be ill fed" and, "It would be unwise to lay down a general diet for all men" (Rorer 1890). Over the course of her career, Mrs. Rorer authored 54 cookbooks, more than 780 articles, and numerous editorials (Cassell 1990). Sara Tyson Rorer was responsible for training the early members of what would become the American Dietetic Association, and she is largely credited for setting the foundations of dietetic education.

Nurse Dietitians

The profession of dietetics has its roots in nursing. Many of the first dietitians were from the nursing profession. Florence Nightingale was credited with contributions to improvement in the food supply and sanitary conditions in hospitals that helped improve the care of the sick during the Crimean War in the mid-1800s (Cooper 1954). Historically, food in U.S. hospitals was monotonous and routine with little variety. One particular account of a New York hospital menu noted that for several days each week, patients were served mush, molasses, and beer for breakfast and supper. Fruits and vegetables were nowhere to be seen and when they were featured in hospital food service, it was usually as a garnish (Winterfeldt Bogle, and Ebro 2014).

History of the American Dietetic Association

The profession of dietetics in the United States formally began with the founding of the American Dietetic Association (ADA). Prior to the establishment of the ADA, the American Home Economics Association served as the professional organization for those working in the areas of food and nutrition. At the first formal meeting of what was to become the ADA, approximately 100 dietitians congregated in Cleveland, Ohio in 1917 for the purpose of "providing an opportunity for the dietitians of the country to come together and meet with the scientific research workers and to see that the feeding of as many people as possible be placed in the hands of women trained to feed them in the best manner known." This Cleveland meeting led to the formal organization of the ADA. Initial topics of discussion at the first meeting included infant feeding, the possibility for the role of dietitians working in hotels and the hospitality industry, collaboration with physicians and "The Dietitian and Her Equipment" (Cassell 1990). Dues were fixed at $1 per year and membership was restricted to those who were trained in the field. The first president of the ADA was Lulu Grace Graves, a former home economics student at the University of Chicago and associate professor of home economics at Iowa State College. At its annual meeting in 1919, Ms. Graves reported on the five categories of membership:

1. Graduates of a two-year course in home economics
2. Graduates of a one-year course in home economics prior to June 1917 and one year of successful experience in dietetics
3. Research workers who had contributed to the advancement of dietetics
4. Practicing physicians in good standing
5. Persons whose special work was allied with dietetics (Graves 1919)

ADA grew in the years following World War I. Dietitians who had collaborated with the armed services during the war "returned with work experience that included the most adverse conditions and with a better understanding of the food habits and the nutritional status of the people of other countries" (Barber 1959). Dietitians began to work in government service, teaching hospitals, and academic institutions. The association appointed chairs for individual sections of practice, including:

- *Dieto-thearpy:* Aiding hospital dietitians who oversaw the preparation of special orders or were preparing the diets in a metabolism ward. The first Chair was Margaret Sawyer, American Red Cross, Washington, DC.
- *Administration:* Of interest to the administrative dietitian who was responsible for supervising the work of culinary departments in hospitals and other establishments, commercial enterprises, and lunchrooms. The first Chair was Emma Smedley, Director of School Lunchrooms, Philadelphia.
- *Teaching:* Provided assistance to dietitians in education who taught student nurses and future dietitians. The first Chair

was Katherine Fisher of Teachers' College of Columbia
University, New York.

- *Social welfare:* Appealed to the interests of the social welfare
  or field dietitian, working in social service agencies, through
  dispensaries or in private consultation. The first Chair was
  Blanche Joseph, Michael Reese Hospital Dispensary,
  Chicago (Cassell 1990).

By 1927, the organization had 1,200 members and its headquarters
were located in Chicago, as they still are today. The *Journal of the American
Dietetic Association* was first published in 1925, distributing four
issues a year and covering topics such as hospital food service, personnel
and management issues, and special diets with a focus on diets for diabetes
(Winterfeldt Bogle, and Ebro 2014).

Leaders of the Profession

In addition to Sarah Tyson Rorer, America's first dietitian, other women
played influential roles in the nascent days of dietetics:

- Ellen H. Richards led the home economics movement and
  was an early leader in the field of dietetics.
- Lulu Graves served as the first president of the ADA and
  started a training course for dietitians at Cornell University.
- Lenna Frances Cooper was an early ADA member and
  president and directed the School of Home Economics at
  Battle Creek Health Care Institution in Michigan, later
  going on to serve on the staff of the U.S. surgeon general in
  Washington, DC.
- Ruth Wheeler first outlined the requirements for a training
  course for student dietitians.
- Mary E. Barber was an ADA president who acted as a food
  consultant in 1941 to aid in the feeding of 1.5 million
  soldiers during World War II. She also edited the first
  official history of the ADA.

- Mary Schwartz Rose established the Department of Nutrition at Columbia University and led nutrition research and nutrition education initiatives.
- Mary P. Huddleston edited the ADA journal from 1927 to 1946 and an annual award is presented each year by the Academy of Nutrition and Dietetics (AND, formerly the ADA) for the author of the best article published in the association's journal in the previous year.
- Anna Boller Beach served as the first executive secretary of the ADA in 1923, was eventually the president, and acted as historian after that (Cassell 1990), (Winterfeldt Bogle, and Ebro 2014).

Developments in the Profession of Dietetics

Minimum requirements for practicing dietitians were established as far back as 1919. Initially, two years of college was recommended. This was later was changed to a four-year requirement (or two-year for institutional managers). Rigorous and thorough nutrition science education has always been a core foundation of dietetics practice.

Continuing Professional Education

Continuing education became a core of the dietitian's practice when dietetics was registered as an accredited profession in the 1960s. The requirement is that 75 hours of continuing education be obtained in every five-year accreditation cycle. As a way to streamline the continuing education process, the Commission on Dietetic Registration (CDR) introduced the Professional Development Portfolio (PDP) to its members to aid in their attaining 75 hours of quality and meaningful continuing education for every five-year cycle.

The PDP allows RDNs and DTRs to identify their own unique learning needs and to map out a continuing education path to meeting these goals. The underlying principle of the PDP process is that "effective continuing professional education (CPE) involves more than information transfer alone," and the PDP process was designed and implemented to "promote lifelong learning and continuing professional competence while providing [registered dietitian nutritionists] with the tools to achieve these aims." The PDP tool allows practitioners to analyze circumstances, requirements, and essential practice competencies within the profession, create and execute an individualized continuing education activity, and to evaluate the success of incorporating CPE in one's professional life (CDR, 2015). The PDP also helps professionals meet the Joint Commission on Accreditation of Healthcare Organizations (JCAH) standards and meet state licensure requirements. It also serves as a tool for career development.

National Nutrition Month

In addition to augmenting knowledge through continuing education among the membership base, the Academy of Nutrition and Dietetics (formerly the American Dietetic Association) has also initiated numerous programs aimed at educating the general population about nutrition. What was originally termed "Dietitian's Week" has evolved into a month-long event each March called National Nutrition Month (NNM). NNM is a nutrition education and information campaign sponsored annually by the Academy of Nutrition and Dietetics. The campaign is designed to highlight the importance of making informed food choices, and to assist individuals and groups in developing sound eating and physical activity habits. Additionally, NNM also serves to promote AND and its members to the public and media as the most valuable and credible sources of timely, scientifically based food and nutrition information (AND, 2015b). More information about the National Nutrition Month campaign and associated education and promotional materials can be found at www.nationalnutritionmonth.org.

Evidence Analysis Library

The Evidence Analysis Library (EAL) is a "synthesis of the best, most relevant nutritional research on important dietetic practice questions housed within an accessible, online, user-friendly library" (AND, 2015a). Launched in 2004, the EAL employs an objective and transparent methodology for assessing food and nutrition-related science. To date, there are nearly 40 projects in various stages that practitioners and researchers alike fall back on as evidence for their practice or work. For each of the nutrition project topics, EAL provides the following resources for practitioners:

- Bibliographies of the research on a given topic
- Conclusion statements providing concise statements of the collective research on a given question
- Grades for each conclusion statement—this provides a way for practitioners to determine how certain we can be of the conclusion statement based on the quality and extensiveness of the supporting evidence
- Evidence summaries that are brief narrative overviews to synthesize the major research findings on a given topic, including overview tables
- Worksheets on every research study analyzed that yield considerable and detailed information on the major findings, methodology and quality of each study.
- Additional recommendations, recommendation strength and narrative, algorithms and links to evidence are provided to complete the transparent and thorough nature of the project (AND, 2015).

American Dietetic Association Name Change

In 2012 the American Dietetic Association changed its name to the Academy of Nutrition and Dietetics. Although the American Dietetic Association had been a recognizable institution for 95 years, the new name was adopted "in order to progress and meet the needs of the changing field of nutrition." Adding the word "academy" highlights the strong science background and emphasizes the academic expertise of its members, who are mostly registered dietitian nutritionists. The organization chose to include the word "nutrition" in the name to communicate members' aptitude for translating nutrition science into easily understandable information. Retaining the word "dietetics" is a tribute to the history of the profession, a "history founded in food and science-based practice." According to the Academy, "Our name communicates who we are and what we do. We are the nutrition experts—the Academy of Nutrition and Dietetics" (AND, 2012).

References

Academy of Nutrition and Dietetics. *About the Evidence Analysis Library.* 2015. http://www.andeal.org/about (accessed October 13, 2015).

___. *Evidence Analysis Library.* 2015. http://www.eatrightpro.org /resources/research/evidence-based-resources/evidence-analysis-library (accessed October 13, 2015).

___. *National Nutrition Month.* 2015. http://www.nationalnutrition month.org/nnm/ (accessed October 13, 2015).

___ *Why the Academy Changed its Name.* 2012. http://www.eatrightpro .org/resource/leadership/board-of-directors/strategic-plan/why-the-academy-changed-its-name (accessed October 13, 2015).

American Dietetic Association. *A New Look at the Profession of Dietetics. Report of the 1984 Study Commission on Dietetics.* Chicago: The American Dietetic Association, 1985, 29.

Barber, MI. *History of the American Dietetic Association: 1917-1959.* Philadelphia: J.B. Lippincott, 1959.

Beeuwkes, AM. "The Prevalence of Scurvy among Voyageurs to America 1493-1600." *J Am Diet Assoc* 24 (1948): 300-303.

Carpenter, KJ. "The Discovery of Vitamin C." *Ann Nutr Metab* 61 (2012): 259-264.

Cassell, JA. *Carry the Flame: The History of the American Dietetic Association.* Chicago: The American Dietetic Association, 1990.

Commission on Dietetic Registration. *Professional Development Portfolio.* 2015. https://www.cdrnet.org/pdp/professional-development-portfolio-guide (accessed October 13, 2015).

Cooper, LF. "Florence Nightingale's Contribution to Dietetics." *J Am Diet Assoc,* 1954: 121-127.

Graves, LG. "President's Report: 1918-1919." Read at 1919 ADA meeting, Cincinnati, OH, 1919.

Rorer, ST. "Early dietetics." *J Am Diet Assoc*, 1934: 289-295.

___. "The dietary." *The Dietetic Gazette*, 1890: 7.

Sholly, C. "Our Story: America's first dietitian lived here." *Lebanon Daily News*, April 1, 2013: 1.

Winterfeldt, EA, and ML Bogle. *Nutrition & Dietetics: Practice and Future.* 4th. Jones & Bartlett Learning, 2013.

CHAPTER 3

Nutrition Credentials

Chapter Abstract

If you work in the field of nutrition and dietetics, you will sooner rather than later be asked, "What is the difference between a dietitian and a nutritionist?" The answer is that all dietitians are nutritionists, but not all nutritionists are dietitians. In fact, in some states the term nutritionist means "nothing"—anyone can go around touting her- or himself as a nutritionist. The general public is constantly seeking nutrition advice and oftentimes not from the most reputable of sources. This chapter seeks to highlight the differences in nutrition credentials to raise the awareness about sources of reliable nutrition information.

Registered Dietitian Nutritionist

The registered dietitian nutritionist (RDN) is a food and nutrition expert who maintains the nationally recognized RDN credential. RDNs are also called registered dietitians (RDs). Currently in the United States, there are more than 89,000 RDNs and the variety of arenas in which they work are covered in Chapter 4.

RDN Credential Criteria

Some RDNs may hold additional advanced degrees or certifications in specialized areas of practice. In order to obtain the RDN credential, a RDN must meet the following criteria:

- Successfully complete a minimum of a bachelor's degree at a U.S. regionally accredited university or college with a course work accredited or approved by the Accreditation Council

for Education in Nutrition and Dietetics (ACEND) of the
Academy of Nutrition and Dietetics (AND)

- Successfully complete an ACEND-accredited supervised
  practice program at a health care facility, community
  agency, or a food service corporation or combined with
  undergraduate or graduate studies. Typically, a practice
  program is six to 12 months long
- Pass a national examination administered by the
  Commission on Dietetic Registration (CDR)
- Successfully complete continuing professional education
  requirements to maintain registration (AND 2015c)

The Commission on Dietetic Registration (CDR) is the credential-
ing agency for AND. Whereas membership in AND is voluntary, all
RDNs must pay CDR an annual fee to maintain their credentials. Some
(but not all) states require that RD/RDNs also become licensed dietitians (LDNs).

Undergraduate Studies

One of the requirements for obtaining the RDN credential is a Baccalaureate degree granted by a U.S. regionally accredited college or university or
foreign equivalent (AND, 2015a). Students must also complete an
ACEND-accredited didactic program in dietetics. Information about
didactic programs in dietetics can be found on the ACEND website available at http://www.eatrightacend.org/ACEND/content.aspx?id=10905.

Supervised Practice—Dietetic Internship

Upon completion of undergraduate studies, those interested in pursuing
the RDN credential must complete supervised practice requirements. This
may be accomplished through either an accredited dietetic internship program or an accredited coordinated program. Both require instruction with
a minimum of 1,200 hours of supervised practice and offer the opportunity for the achievement of knowledge and performance requirement for
entry-level dietitians. The difference between the dietetic internship and

the coordinated program is that the coordinated program allows students to complete their supervised practice while also enrolled in their undergraduate or graduate program, whereas the dietetic internship is done separately and after completion of the Didactic Program in Dietetics (DPD) requirements. The ACEND website contains information about accredited dietetic internship programs and coordinated programs. Internships or coordinated programs differ in their requirements (distance versus local rotations) and length (from six months to two years), although all require at least 1,200 hours minimum of supervised practice.

Individual Supervised Practice Pathways (ISPPs)

In 2011, AND announced the development of the Individual Supervised Practice Pathways or ISPPs (pronounced "ispeys"). These were created to give students more options for educational experiences that will allow them to be eligible to sit for the registration exam. ISPPs are essentially alternate pathways that add supervised practice capacity through ACEND-accredited dietetics programs while allowing students protections that were previously missing from former, unaccredited models. These pathways align DPD students who have verification statements to obtain supervised practice. More information about this option can be found at http://www.eatrightacend.org/ACEND/content.aspx?id=6442485529.

Registration Examination for Dietitians

Upon completion of the education and supervised practice requirements, an individual may advance to sit for the national registration examination for dietitians. This exam is computer based and is administered by CDR. It is designed to evaluate a dietitian's ability to perform at the entry level. The registration examination includes questions on topics such as the principles of dietetics, nutrition care for individuals and groups, management of food and nutrition programs, services and food service systems.

Continuing Professional Education

After passing the one-time national registration examination, RDNs must complete at least 75 hours of continuing professional education in every five-year reporting cycle. The purpose of continuing professional education (CPE) is to ensure that these credentialed nutrition professionals are staying abreast of scientific changes in the field and maintaining professional competence. CDR has developed the Professional Development Portfolio (PDP) that serves as a process for CPE to promote lifelong learning and continuing professional competence. More information about CPE and the PDP can be found in Chapter 5 and online at https://www.cdrnet.org.

Specialist Board Certification

The Commission on Dietetic Registration offers Board Certification as a Specialist in Pediatric Nutrition, Renal Nutrition, Gerontological Nutrition, Oncology Nutrition, and Sports Dietetics. Obtaining specialist board certification is done in addition and on top of the requirements of the RDN credential. Specialist board certification indicates the individual has documented practice experience and has successfully completed an examination in his or her specialty area.

Board Certified Specialist in Pediatric Nutrition (CSP)

RDNs who work in pediatric nutrition settings may wish to validate their expertise by obtaining the Board Certified Specialist in Pediatric Nutrition (CSP) credential. The exam is administered by CDR twice a year. Qualified individuals who sit for the exam are well versed in pediatric nutrition conditions such as congenital heart disease, cystic fibrosis, diabetes, developmental disabilities, dyslipidemia/hyperlipidemia, failure to thrive, food intolerances/allergies, gastrointestinal disorders/problems, lactation, healthy infants/children, obesity/overweight, oral feeding disorders, parenteral nutrition, premature infants, pulmonary disorders, specific nutrient deficiencies, tube feeding, and vegetarianism (CDR, 2012).

Board Certified Specialist in Renal Nutrition (CSR)

RDNs who work in kidney (renal) disease and nutrition settings may wish to validate their expertise by obtaining the Board Certified Specialist in Renal Nutrition (CSR) credential. The exam is administered by CDR twice a year. Qualified individuals who sit for the exam are well versed in renal nutrition conditions such as chronic kidney disease, kidney transplantation, mineral bone disorders, end-stage renal disease, hemodialysis, peritoneal dialysis, fluid management, renal laboratory data, and national renal guidelines and standards (CDR, 2012). Renal nutrition practice that qualifies the individual for specialty practice experience includes working directly with adults and/or children with acute or chronic renal dysfunction or failure, under treatment by kidney transplantation, dialysis, or other modalities in a variety of settings (home, hospitals, other treatment centers, etc.) or indirectly as documented by management, education, or research practice linked specifically to renal nutrition (CDR, 2015).

Board Certified Specialist in Gerontological Nutrition (CSG)

RDNs who work with older adults in gerontological nutrition settings may wish to validate their expertise by obtaining the Board Certified Specialist in Gerontological Nutrition (CSG) credential. The exam is administered by CDR twice a year. Qualified individuals who sit for the exam are well versed in the nutritional care of older adults as it pertains to the aging process. Topics of expertise of these practitioners includes nutrition assessment, hydration status, metabolic and physical changes associated with aging, risk factors associated with socioeconomic status, social and psychological factors, identifying nutrient imbalances, food/drug interactions, nutrition diagnosis, and federal regulations and nutrition program requirements that relate to nutrition care of older adults in facility and community settings (CDR, 2015).

Board Certified Specialist in Oncology Nutrition (CSO)

RDNs who work with cancer patients may wish to validate their expertise by obtaining the Board Certified Specialist in Oncology Nutrition (CSO) credential. The exam is administered by CDR twice a year. Qualified individuals who sit for the exam are well versed in the nutritional care of cancer patients. Topics of expertise of these practitioners includes specific types of cancer, treatment effects and impact on nutritional status, signs and symptoms of nutrition problems, evidence-based nutrition interventions for use in cancer care, nutrition support, and cancer risk reduction. RDNs who work directly with individuals who are at risk for or diagnosed with any type of malignancy or pre-malignant condition in a variety of health care settings, or who are indirectly involved through roles in management, education, industry, and research practice linked specifically to oncology nutrition may be considered as having specialty practice experience and be qualified to obtain this credential (CDR, 2015).

Board Certified Specialist in Sports Dietetics (CSSD)

RDNs who work in sports dietetics may wish to validate their expertise by obtaining the Board Certified Specialist in Sports Dietetics (CSSD) credential. The exam is administered by CDR twice a year. Specialty Practice Experience for interested CSSDs includes working as an RDN for a minimum of two years applying evidence-based nutrition knowledge in exercise and sports. CSSDs assess, educate, and counsel athletes and active individuals. They design, implement, and manage safe and effective nutrition strategies that enhance lifelong health, fitness, and performance (CDR, 2015).

Graduate Degrees in Nutrition

In 2012, AND proposed raising the minimum education requirement for entry-level RD to a graduate degree from an ACEND-accredited program. Currently, the entry-level requirement is a baccalaureate degree. The recommendation for graduate degree will take place beginning in the year 2024.

It is estimated that 45 percent of RDNs have a graduate degree and 4 percent have doctoral degrees (AND, 2005). According to the 2011 AND Compensation and Benefits survey, RDNs who have a graduate degree can expect to earn $2.41 more per hour (for a total of approximately $5,000 more per year) than RDNs with a bachelor's degree (Ward 2012). RDNs may augment their nutrition expertise with graduate degrees in any one of a number of subjects. Some RDNs have Master of Science (MS), Master of Public Health (MPH), Master of Education (MEd), Master of Public Policy (MPP), or Master of Business Administration (MBA). Some students who enter graduate study programs may already have obtained the RDN credential, or may be working towards their RDN credential while concurrently working towards their graduate degree. Students interested in pursuing nutrition-related graduate studies either in conjunction with a coordinated program in dietetics or dietetic internship may be interested in researching ACEND-accredited programs listed online at http://www.eatrightacend.org/ACEND/content.aspx?id=73. It may also be the case that an individual has completed a graduate degree in a nutrition-related topic but does not have the RDN credential. These nutrition professionals may work in the fields of public health nutrition, nutrition research, nutrition education, or private practice. Generally, a graduate without the RDN credential does not work in a clinical setting with direct patient care, as those positions tend to require the RDN credential.

Dietetic Technician, Registered

Dietetic technicians, registered (DTRs), also often called Diet Techs, are "educated and trained at the technical level of nutrition and dietetics practice for the delivery of safe, culturally competent, quality food and nutrition services" (AND, 2015c)." DTRs work under the supervision of RDNs when they are employed in direct patient or nutrition client care in practice areas such as hospitals, clinics, skilled nursing facilities, hospices, home health care programs and research facilities. DTRs are qualified to conduct patient and client screens, gather data, and to perform assigned tasks to assist RDNs in the provision of medical nutrition therapy (MNT).

DTRs are nationally credentialed food and nutrition practitioners. In order to obtain the DTR credential, a DTR must meet the following criteria:

- Successfully complete a Dietetic Technician Program accredited by ACEND that includes 450 hours of supervised practice experience in various community-based programs, health care and food service facilities
- Successfully complete at least a two year associate's degree at a U.S. regionally accredited college or university
- Successfully complete Registration Examination for Dietetic Technicians
- Complete 50 hours of continuing education every five years (AND, 2015a).

There is also an option for individuals who have already completed a Baccalaureate degree from a U.S. regionally accredited college or university or foreign equivalent and who have completed an ACEND Didactic Program in Dietetics to sit for the registration exam.

Currently in the United States, the number of RDNs far surpasses that of DTRs. As of 2015, there were 5,461 DTRs in the United States as compared to 93,946 RDNs (CDR, 2015). Although the number of DTRs is small, there are many opportunities for DTRs. These include:

- Schools, day care centers, correctional facilities, restaurants, health care facilities, corporations, and hospitals; DTRs manage employees, purchase and prepare food, and maintain budgets within food service operations.
- Women, Infant, Children (WIC) programs, public health agencies, Meals on Wheels and other community health programs; DTRs assist RDNs with the implementation of programs and presentation of classes for the public.
- Health clubs, weight management clinics, and community health and wellness centers; DTRs help to educate clients about the connection between food, fitness, and health.

- Food companies, contract food management companies, or food vending distribution operations; DTRs develop menus, conduct nutrient analysis and data collection, and oversee food service sanitation and food safety (AND, 2015).

According to the AND's 2009 Dietetic Compensation and Benefits Survey, half of all DTRs in the U.S. have been working in the field for less than five years. Stated salaries are between $33,800 and $37,700 per year; however, salary levels vary by region, employment setting, geographical location, and scope of responsibility, and supply of DTRs (AND, 2015).

Nutritionists and Other Nutrition Credentials

Unlike the registered dietitian (RD) or registered dietitian nutritionist (RDN) credential, the title "nutritionist" is much less regulated. In the United States, some states require additional licensure in order to carry the title "nutritionist" while others may not. A person who holds a master's degree may be called a nutritionist, although the title nutritionist is also used loosely by a variety of other people, who may or may not have a fundamental knowledge base and demonstrated expertise in the field of nutrition science. The next chapter outlines opportunities for employment in the field of nutrition and also includes information about where non-RDN nutrition professionals may work.

Nutrition in Primary Care

The dearth of nutrition education in medical and primary care curricula is well established and is certainly lamentable. Only 25 percent of accredited medical schools in the United States offer their students a dedicated nutrition class, and only 27 percent of those institutions meet the minimum 25 hours of nutrition education recommended by the National Academy of Sciences. Despite the public's increasing interest in nutrition and society's coincident, and ironically spiking obesity rates, these medical nutrition education numbers are actually on the decline

(Adams, Kohlmeier and Zeisel 2010). As the general population grows, the more we need practitioners educated in nutrition, the less likely we are to be actually getting them. With approximately two-thirds of the American adult population being overweight or obese and the majority of our primary care providers having never taken a nutrition course, the gaping knowledge deficit about diet and disease becomes more pronounced. One analysis of more than 10,000 patient visits found that the odds of receiving counseling for diet and nutrition, exercise, or weight loss from a physician actually declined by 22 percent from the period of 1995/1996 to 2001/2002 (McAlpine and Wilson 2007).

Why do primary care practitioners shy away from educating patients about the relationship between their food choices and health status? There are a myriad of reasons, or perhaps excuses, in today's health care environment. Among them, time constraints, scarcity of training resources, lack of reimbursement for nutrition counseling, questionable nutrition intervention studies, patient noncompliance, and even practitioners' own weight insecurities may all contribute. Recall the story of Dr. Terry Bennett in New Hampshire, whose patient filed a complaint with the state Board of Medicine after he told her she was obese and that it was hurting her health (ABC Good Morning America 2005). Even fear of litigation can limit one's willingness to talk about weight.

But it turns out that even talking about weight can jump-start positive behaviors. One recent study looked at the effect of a physician telling overweight and obese people that they were overweight. Those who were overweight (BMI of 25 or greater) or obese (BMI of 30 or greater) had an increased likelihood of having attempted to lose weight in the previous year if their doctor had told them that they were overweight. The problem was only 45.2 percent of individuals with a BMI of 25 or greater and 66.4 percent of those with a BMI of 30 or greater reported being told by a physician that they were overweight (Post et al. 2011). Without making light of it, we are essentially ignoring the elephant in the room.

Perhaps above all of these reasons, it is a lack of confidence in nutrition counseling techniques that is the most likely culprit paralyzing even the best of practitioners' intentions. In one survey of over 500 American physicians, 36 percent said they were knowledgeable about weight management techniques, but only 3 percent were confident that those coun-seling techniques succeed in their practice (Castaldo et al. 2005). And it's not just American primary care providers (PCPs). In Canada, 82.3 percent of physicians surveyed in one study reported their formal nutri-tion training in medical school to be inadequate, and nearly all of those physicians surveyed identified a lack of time and compensation as the largest barriers to providing nutrition guidance (Wynn et al. 2010). Euro-pean health care professionals do not fare well either, with numerous studies concluding that knowledge about the prevention and treatment of malnutrition is poor (Ray et al. 2012), (Kafatos 2009), (Nightingale and Reeves 1999).

There is less data regarding the nutrition education and nutrition counseling competency of advanced practice nurses. Of the top 10 Fam-ily Nurse Practitioner and top 16 Adult Nurse Practitioner graduate school programs ranked by U.S. News and World Report in 2011, only one of the 16 different schools offer a stand-alone nutrition course (U.S. News & World Report 2011). While nutrition is no doubt included as a part of other classes within the advanced practice nursing curriculum spectrum, the lack of attention to the importance of directly addressing nutrition-related concerns and the system-wide lack of development of nutrition counseling skills for practitioners is concerning. The problem is not limited to advanced practice nurses, as all PCPs are likely under-trained to address nutrition and weight related problems. These limita-tions also spill over into the territory of herbal and dietary supplements.

Patients and clients are increasingly turning to the use of and asking about the effectiveness and safety of dietary supplements and herbal remedies. One recent study analyzed physicians', APNs', pharmacists', and dietitians' knowledge, attitudes, and practices of herbs and other dietary supplements. The average score on knowledge was 10 out of 20 points, confidence was 4 out of 10 possible points, and average commu-nication score was 1.4 out of 4 possible points (Kemper et al. 2003).

In today's health care environment, primary care practitioners often do not have the luxury of spending a leisurely hour or two with each patient, carefully combing through their food intake patterns and gently broaching the topic of weight, nutrition, and health. The breakneck pace of primary care requires multi-tasking, prioritizing, and triaging. When it comes to talking nutrition, a practitioner's modus operandi is more likely to be *reactive* than *proactive*. Think about a single mother who brings her sick infant along with his healthy older brother to a clinic appointment. Mom is concerned about her baby getting better, and she is not likely to focus on her sedentary, video-game playing, overweight school-age son with prediabetes and high blood pressure who happens to be munching on potato chips while in the clinic.

It is understandable that not every patient encounter presents an appropriate time to discuss nutrition; however, practitioners can learn to recognize nutrition teaching moments, screen for nutrition risk, implement brief assessment tools, and identify and refer to other community nutrition resources that will help those patients who need education, information, and assistance. Increasingly, the majority of patients need these resources. Ignoring their needs is not a viable option. It is up to the front-line practitioners to make nutrition a priority and to bridge the knowledge gap about diet and disease for our patients and clients.

Although most medical schools include nutrition in their curriculum, the vast majority of practicing physicians have never taken a dedicated nutrition course. There are some physicians, however, who are specialists in nutrition, and they will likely have the Physician Nutrition Specialist credential. A Physician Nutrition Specialist (PNS) is an expert in clinical nutrition who is committed to "applying rigorous, evidence-based medicine to clinical nutrition practice." PNS practitioners have earned a Medical Doctor (MD), Doctor of Osteopathy (DO), or an equivalent degree and have usually completed residency programs in the specialties of internal medicine, pediatrics, family medicine, or general surgery (NBPNS, 2015).

Beware of Unqualified Individuals

Despite the numerous avenues available to demonstrate expertise in nutrition and obtain legitimate credentials, our current health care and weight loss environment has no shortage of quacks and hucksters working for ulterior motives. The Internet is rife with misinformation and misleading claims about foods and supplements. A very valuable resource is the National Institutes of Health's website "How to Evaluate Health Information on the Internet: Questions and Answers" available at https://ods.od.nih.gov/Health_Information/How_To_Evaluate_Health_Information_on_the_Internet_Questions_and_Answers.aspx. The key points are that a website should clearly identify the original source of the information and health-related websites should give information about the medical credentials of the people who have prepared or reviewed the material on the site. Writing about "Where to Get Professional Nutrition Advice" on his website Quackwatch, the retired physician and cofounder of the National Council Against Health Fraud, Stephen Barrett, MD, advises readers to steer clear of the following:

- Anyone who says that everyone needs vitamin supplements to be sure they get enough. Most people can get all the vitamins they need by eating sensibly.
- Anyone who suggests that most diseases are caused by faulty nutrition. Although some diseases are diet related, most are not.
- Anyone who suggests that large doses of vitamins are effective against a large number of diseases and conditions. That is simply untrue.
- Anyone who suggests hair analysis as a basis for determining the body's nutritional state or for recommending vitamins and minerals. Hair analysis is not reliable for this purpose.
- Anyone who claims that a wide variety of symptoms and diseases are caused by "hidden food allergies."
- Anyone who uses a computer-scored "nutrient deficiency test" as the basis for prescribing vitamins. There are valid ways that computers can be used for dietary analysis. But those used for recommending vitamins are programmed to recommend them for everyone.
- All practitioners—licensed or not—who sell vitamins in their offices. Scientific nutritionists do not sell vitamins. Unscientific practitioners often do—usually at a considerable profit (Barrett 2012).

References

ABC Good Morning America. 2005. *Doctor Reprimanded for Calling Patient Fat.* New York, NY.

Academy of Nutrition and Dietetics. 2005. *2005 Compensation and Benefits Survey.* Chicago: Academy of Nutrition and Dietetics.

Academy of Nutrition and Dietetics. 2015. *Becoming a Dietetic Technician, Registered.* www.eatrightpro.org/resource/about-us/what-is-an-rdn-and-dtr/what-is-a-dietetic-technician-registered/becoming-a-dietetic-technician-registered, (accessed September 30, 2015).

Academy of Nutrition and Dietetics. 2015a. *Registration Eligibility Requirements for Dietitians.* www.cdrnet.org/certifications/registration-eligibility-requirements-for-dietitians, (accessed October 7, 2015).

Academy of Nutrition and Dietetics. 2015b. *What Is a Dietic Technician, Registered?* www.eatrightpro.org/resources/about-us/what-is-an-rdn-and-dtr/what-is-a-dietetic-technician-registered, (accessed September 30, 2015).

Academy of Nutrition and Dietetics. 2015c. *What Is a Registered Dietitian Nutritionist?* www.eatrightpro.org/resources/about-us/what-is-an-rdn-and-dtr/what-is-a-registered-dietitian-nutritionist, (accessed September 30, 2015).

Adams, K.M., M. Kohlmeier, and S.H. Zeisel. September, 2010. "Nutrition Education in U.S. Medical Schools: Latest Update of a National Survey." *Academic Medicine* 85, no. 9, pp. 1537–42.

Barrett, S. 2012. *Where to Get Professional Nutrition Advice.* www.quackwatch.org/04ConsumerEducation/nutritionist.html, (accessed October 7, 2015).

Castaldo, J., J. Nester, T. Wasser, T. Masiado, M. Rossi, M. Young, J.J. Napolitano, J.S. Schwartc. April, 2005. "Physician Attitudes Regarding Cardiovascular Risk Reduction: The Gaps Between Clinical Importance, Knowledge, and Effectiveness." *Disease Management* 8, no. 2, pp. 93–105.

Commission on Dietetic Registration. 2012a. *Board Certified Specialist in Renal Nutrition Certification Examination Content Outline.* www.cdrnet.org/vault/2459/web/files/RenalNutritionContentOutline 2005.pdf, (accessed September 30, 2015).

Commission on Dietetic Registration. 2012b. *Pediatric Nutrition Conent Outline.* www.cdrnet.org/vault/2459/web/files/CDR%20Peds%20Content%20Outline.pdf, (accessed September 30, 2015).

Commission on Dietetic Registration. 2015a. *Gerontological Nutrition Examination Content Outline.* admin.cdrnet.org/vault/2459/web/files /CSGContentOutline.pdf, (accessed September 30, 2015).

Commission on Dietetic Registration. 2015b. *RDN or RD and NDTR or DTR Credentials.* www.cdrnet.org/#, (accessed September 30, 2015).

Commission on Dietetic Registration. 2015c. *Specialty Practice Experience.* www.cdrnet.org/certifications/specialty-practice-experience#gerontological, (accessed September 30, 2015).

Kafatos, A. May, 2009."Is Clinical Nutrition Teaching Needed in Medical Schools." *Annals of Nutrition and Metabolism* 54, no. 2, pp. 129–30.

Kemper, K.J., A. Amata-Kynvi, L. Dvorkin, J.S. Whelan, A. Woolf, R.C. Samuels, P. Hibberd. May–June, 2003. "Herbs and Other Dietary Supplements: Healthcare Professionals' Knowledge, Attitudes, and Practices." *Alternative Therapies in Health and Medicine* 9, no. 3, pp. 42–9.

McAlpine, D.D. and A.R. Wilson. April, 2007."Trends in Obesity-related Counseling in Primary Care: 1995–2004." *Medical Care* 45, no. 4, pp. 322–9.

National Board of Physician Nutrition Specialists. 2015. *What Is a Physician Nutrition Specialist?* www.nutritioncare.org/nbpns/, (accessed October 7, 2015).

Nightingale, J.M. and J. Reeves. February, 1999. "Knowledge about the Assessment and Management of Undernutrition: A Pilot Questionnaire in a UK Teaching Hospital." *Clinical Nutrition* 18, no. 1, pp. 23–7.

Post, R.E., A.G., 3rd Mainous, S.H. Gregorie, M.E. Knoll, V.A. Diaz, and S.K. Saxena. February, 2011. "The Influence of Physician Acknowledgment of Patients' Weight Status on Patient Perceptions of Overweight and Obesity in the United States." *Archives of Internal Medicine* 171, no. 4, pp. 316–21.

Ray, S., R. Udumyan, M. Rajput-Ray, B. Thompson, K.M. Lodge, P. Douglas, P. Sharma, R. Broughton, S. Smart, R. Wilson, S. Gillam,

M.J. van der Es, I. Fisher, and J. Gandy. February, 2012. "Evaluation of a Novel Nutrition Education Intervention for Medical Students from across England." *BMJ Open* 2, no. 1, p. e000417.

US News & World Report. 2011. "Nurse Practitioner: Adult." *Education: Graduate Schools.*

Ward, B. January, 2012. "Compensation and Benefits Survey 2011: Moderate Growth in Registered Dietitian and Dietetic Technician, Registered, Compensation in the Past 2 Years." *Journal of the Academy of Nutrition and Dietetics* 112, no. 1, pp. 29–40.

Wynn, K., J.D. Trudeau, K. Taunton, M .Gowans, and I. Scott. March, 2010."Nutrition in Primary Care: Current Practices, Attitudes, and Barriers." *Canadian Family Physician* 56, no. 3, pp. E109–16.

CHAPTER 4

Career Opportunities in Nutrition and Dietetics

Chapter Abstract

Deciding to become a credentialed nutrition practitioner opens up a wide world of career opportunities. Some individuals may go into the field with a desire to help prevent and manage disease, whereas others may be interested in food service management. Still others may want to work with athletes, people with eating disorders, business entities, research endeavors, or any number of underserved populations. Suffice it to say that wherever there is food, there is a need for a nutrition professional. This chapter outlines the various places of employment and typical compensation for professionals working in the field of nutrition and dietetics. The information provided pertains primarily to registered dietitian nutritionists (RDNs) and dietetic technicians, registered (DTRs). Although opportunities do exist for those working in nutrition without these credentials, there is much less employment data available due to a lack of other national credentials and the variation in licensure from state to state.

Places of Employment

RDNs are employed in a variety of settings that include health care, business and industry, community and public health, education, research, government agencies and private practice. Many health care specific work environments do require that the individual be credentialed as an RDN, although there are other settings where one can gain experience in nutrition or work without a credential, although opportunities may be limited.

Hospitals, Clinics, or Other Health Care Facilities

It comes as no surprise that the majority of nutrition professionals with the RDN credential practice in the health care setting. Many people go into the profession with a desire to help others make positive food choices that can help prevent, manage, or in some cases even contribute to a cure maladies. RDNs who work in hospitals, clinics, or other health care facilities often function as part of an interdisciplinary team who intend to at treating the whole individual. These nutrition professionals educate patients about nutrition and are trained in the administration of medical nutrition therapy (MNT) in their role in the health care team. There is also a need for credentialed professionals to manage food service operations in health care and correctional facilities, and these people may be employed in everything from food purchasing, to budgeting, to preparation of food, and management of food service staff.

Most RDNs gain initial exposure to clinical dietetics through their supervised practice that is a mandatory part of the preparation for the profession. Dietetic interns spend time working under a preceptor RDNs to learn about the roles of screening and interviewing patients and clients, identifying nutrition risk and ascribing nutrition diagnosis, planning and implementing nutrition interventions, and tracking outcomes and monitoring the effectiveness of these interventions. The opportunities in the clinical setting may be in the acute, inpatient care side, where RDNs may work in a nutrition support team in the intensive care unit (ICU), or in the outpatient setting providing individual nutrition or group counseling on diet and nutrition. Additional health care facility work may include long-term care (nursing homes) or adult day health care centers. These practitioners may desire to obtain additional specialist credentials in their area of expertise such as oncology, renal, pediatric, sports, or geriatric nutrition (see Chapter 2 for board certification in dietetics opportunities).

Sports Nutrition

Interest in sports dietitians is certainly growing as athletes, coaches, and wellness professionals increasingly recognize and value the link between food, fitness, and health. Many RDNs who work in the sports nutrition field also become board certified specialists in sports dietetics (CSSD). This is considered to be the "premier professional sports nutrition credential in the United States." According to the Sports, Cardiovascular, and Wellness Nutrition (SCAN) dietetic practice group of the Academy of Nutrition and Dietetics, "sports dietitians are experienced registered dietitians who apply evidence-based nutrition knowledge in exercise and sports. They assess, educate, and counsel athletes and active individuals. They design, implement, and manage safe and effective nutrition strategies that enhance lifelong health, fitness, and optimal performance" (Sports, Cardiovascular and Wellness Nutrition (SCAN, 2015). Nutrition professionals with the CSSD certification apply sports nutrition science to support fitness, sport, and athletic performance. Individuals working in sports nutrition may be employed in any of the following areas:

- Athletic performance companies—helping to formulate products or track efficacy of products on athletic populations
- Colleges and universities—working in athletics, student health, campus wellness, and with faculty and staff
- Corporations—focusing on wellness and the food industry
- Health care organization—helping individuals in cardiac rehabilitation or eating disorder treatment centers
- Online nutrition coaching—providing one-on-one or group coaching and counseling
- Professional sports organizations—providing tailored nutrition plans for athletes
- Private practice—counseling patients throughout the lifespan on the importance of optimal nutrition for athletic performance
- U.S. Olympic Committee and training facilities—training current and future Olympic athletes with regard to diet and performance

For more information about sports nutrition and sports dietetics, see the Sports Nutrition information from the SCAN group available at http://www.scandpg.org/sports-nutrition/.

Corporate Wellness Programs

There is a heightened interest in the role of nutrition in prevention of diseases, and only in a few other places will you see more interest in preventing diet-related diseases than in the corporate workplace. America's employers are interested in evidence-based approaches to reduce workplace injury and chronic disease. This presents a unique opportunity for nutrition professionals to help alter the work environment to make it healthier for individuals and groups. Corporate wellness dietitians may be involved in a range of activities, from planning healthier vending campaigns, overseeing cafeteria nutrition labeling initiatives, running health risk screening events or group weight loss challenges, to coordinating group fitness or individual nutrition counseling sessions. Nutrition professionals interested in exploring opportunities in corporate nutrition may be interested in the publication *A Dietitian's Guide to Corporate Health Promotion* published by the Nutrition Entrepreneurs dietetic practice group of the Academy of Nutrition and Dietetics, available at https://nedpg.org/products-services/dietitians-guide-corporate-health-promotion-0.

Food and Nutrition-Related Business and Industries

When you think of employment opportunities in nutrition and dietetics, anywhere there is food, there is a legitimate need for a dietitian. In addition to health, food service and sports nutrition, dietitians also work in food- and nutrition-related business and industries. These private businesses and groups are interested in dietitians who can help translate scientific information about nutrition into useful and practical messages for consumers and thus drive sales. Food manufacturers, health care companies, restaurant chains, weight loss programs, and health technology companies are all potential places of employment for business- and industry-minded dietitians. The Dietitians in Business Communication (DBC) dietetic practice group of the Academy of Nutrition and Dietetics provides information about employment and mentoring opportunities for practitioners interested in this line of work on their website, http://www.dbconline.org.

Food Service Management

Food service professionals span the bridge between nutrition knowledge and food service delivery. These nutrition professionals may run or work in food service operations located in hospitals and clinics, school districts, correctional facilities, colleges and universities, and hotels or restaurants. Nutrition professionals working in food service are usually employed at the management level and may be responsible for menu planning, therapeutic diet considerations, nutrient analysis of menu items, and strategic leadership of staff. For more information about opportunities in this line of work, see the Management in Food and Nutrition Systems, a dietetic practice group of the Academy of Nutrition and Dietetics website at http://www.rdmanager.org/index.php.

Private Practice

Nutrition professionals may decide they are best suited to private practice. Private practitioners usually provide counseling to individuals or groups in an outpatient office setting. The private practitioner's office may be a standalone operation or affiliated with a physician's office. Dietitians working in private practice may specialize in weight loss, pediatric or childhood nutrition, cardiovascular or diabetes management or may have unique specialty areas such as advanced knowledge of food allergens, development of meal plans, eating disorder management, or weight loss. These professionals may choose to accept insurance plans and bill insurance for reimbursement of services or may take private-paying patients only.

In addition to providing individual nutrition counseling, there are many other ways for a nutrition professional to be employed in private practice. The practitioners area of expertise may involve consulting with food companies for menu labeling, freelance writing or authoring of publications, providing consultant nutrition services in long-term care or adult day health care facilities, or contracting with home health care companies, media outlets, or other business entities. Although the majority of private practice dietitians work in a traditional face-to-face office setting, the advent of telehealth, online education, and web-based media outlets affords a great variety of opportunity for expanding the reach of the private practitioner.

Media

The media landscape is changing—and where consumers are going for health information is also evolving. Media dietitians work to help communicate accurate, credible, and timely food and nutrition information to the public and media (AND, 2015). Many media experts work in traditional outlets such as television and print publications. They may be involved in directing or organizing television segments, writing or contributing to articles that highlight new products, summarizing emerging research, or providing commentary on current dietary practices and trends. With the advent of social media, the need for media-savvy dietitians who can clearly and concisely translate complicated scientific matters for the general public is heightened. The Pew Research Center's Pew Internet Project estimates that 72 percent of Internet users say they have looked online for health information within the past year (PRC, 2014). Media dietitians help companies, public relations firms, and various organizations and institutions craft messages about food and nutrition for specific audiences. They may host podcasts, write nutrition blogs, contribute to monthly television segments, or participate in media tours to highlight a wide range of food and health related issues.

Community and Public Health Settings

Another arena for employment consideration in nutrition is that of the community or public health setting. Dietitians can work as a dietitian officer in the U.S. Public Health Service (USPHS) Commissioned Corps, working to improve health and quality of life. These professionals manage nutrition education programs for patients, providers, and the public and conduct research to help improve national and global nutrition (HHS, 2014). Other public health or community opportunities include working in nutrition assistance programs like the USDA's Special Supplemental Nutrition Program for Women, Infants, and Children (WIC), the Supplemental Nutrition Assistance Program (SNAP, formerly known as Food Stamps), public health offices or community clinics. Work may range from individual counseling to programming, education, and development of resources for communities. Some public health or community health dietitians may have also earned an undergraduate or graduate degree in public health and specialize in planning, implementing, and evaluating various public health nutrition programs for local, state, and federal municipalities.

Universities and Medical Centers

Nutrition professionals with advanced degrees may be interested in teaching future practitioners about nutrition. These educators are usually employed at colleges and universities and may be clinical or classroom instructors or faculty, administrators, or researchers. Some university-based professionals will also be affiliated with medical centers and may conduct research programs or patient clinics. They may be responsible for educating future dietetics practitioners, nurses, physician's assistants, dentists, medical doctors, or nurse practitioners.

Research Areas

Opportunities exist for nutrition professionals to contribute to research at the university or academic level, and in the government or the private industry. These nutrition experts may work for food and pharmaceutical companies, hospitals, or colleges and universities. Their work may involve conducting experiments intended to answer critical nutrition questions or to find evidence-based solutions to food-based problems.

International Nutrition Work

There are also opportunities for nutrition professionals to work overseas in development work. These individuals may be employed in emergency nutrition programs, providing food and support for underserved areas ravaged by famine, natural disaster or disease, or displaced due to geopolitical strife. International agencies such as the World Health Organization, World Food Programme (WFP), or the United Nations Children's Fund (UNICEF) have temporary and long-term employment options for internationally-minded individuals. Some nutrition professionals from the United States may get their start in the development sector by serving as Peace Corps Volunteers. The Peace Corps sends American volunteers to "tackle the most pressing needs of people around the world." Their mission is to promote world peace and friendship by fulfilling three goals:

- Help the people of interested countries in meeting their need for trained men and women
- Help promote a better understanding of Americans on the part of the populations served
- Help promote a better understanding of other populations on the part of Americans (USPC, 2014).

Approximately 24 percent of Peace Corps Volunteers work in some health capacity in their host country. Volunteers serve for two years following their in country technical, language and cultural training. To learn more about the opportunities for serving as a Peace Corps Volunteer, visit http://www.peacecorps.gov.

Statistical Data

With regards to place of employment, the 2013 Compensation and Benefits Survey of the Dietetics Profession indicated that 7 percent of practitioners are self-employed, 30 percent work at a for-profit firm, 38 percent work at a nonprofit organization, and 19 percent work for the government (Rogers 2014). Table 4.1 contains more information about the prevalence of dietetics-related employment.

Table 4.1 Prevalence of dietetics-related employment, from Compensation and Benefits Survey of the Dietetics Professions 2013 (Rogers 2014)

	Number of Respondents	Percent in Dietetics
Registered dietitian nutritionist (RDN)	7,783	84%
Dietetic technician, registered (DTR)	1,142	76%
Non-registered professionals	133	60%
Total	9,58	82%

The most common work environment for RDNs is an inpatient acute care facility, with 24 percent of respondents employed there. Twelve percent are employed in an ambulatory or outpatient care facility such as a clinic or doctor's office. This is followed by employment in long-term care, extended care, or assisted living facilities such as a nursing home, at 10 percent. Combined, these top three employment settings encompass almost half of all practicing RDNs. The remainder of professionals work in a variety of other settings, with none representing more than 7 percent of the responding workforce (Rogers 2014).

Although DTRs represent a much smaller percentage of the credentialed workforce, the majority of these professionals work in two settings: 33 percent are employed in inpatient acute care facilities and 27 percent work in long-term care, extended care, or assisted living facilities. Another 8 percent are employed in a community or public health program, with no other setting representing more than 5 percent of DTR employment (Rogers 2014). Table 4.2 highlights the practice area of practicing RDNs and DTRs and Table 4.3 covers the most prevalent positions of RDNs.

Table 4.2 Practice area of practicing RDNs (n = 6,523) and DTRs (n = 866) from the 2013 Compensation and Benefits Survey of the Dietetics Profession (Rogers 2014)

	RDNs	DTRs
Clinical nutrition—acute care/inpatient	32%	44%
Clinical nutrition—ambulatory care	17%	1%
Clinical nutrition—long-term care	8%	13%
Community	11%	11%
Food and nutrition management	12%	19%
Consultation and business	8%	2%
Education and research	6%	2%

Table 4.3 Most prevalent positions among practicing RDNs (n = 6,523) from 2013 Compensation and Benefits Survey of the Dietetics Profession (Rogers 2014)

Clinical dietitian	16%
Clinical dietitian, specialist—renal	3%
Pediatric/neonatal dietitian	3%
Nutrition support dietitian	3%
Outpatient dietitian, general	4%
Outpatient dietitian, specialist—diabetes	4%
Outpatient dietitian, specialist—renal	3%
Clinical dietitian, long-term care	8%
WIC nutritionist	6%
Public health nutritionist	3%
Director of food and nutrition services	5%
Clinical nutrition manager	3%

Who Works in Dietetics

The profession of nutrition and dietetics has historically been and continues to be largely dominated by Caucasian female practitioners. According to the 2013 Compensation and Benefits Survey of the Dietetics Profession, 95 percent of practitioners are female. The median age is 46 years, and 29 percent are 55 or older and 26 percent are under 35. Regarding ethnic identification, 4 percent are of Hispanic heritage and 9 percent of respondents indicated they are a race other than white (5 percent Asian, 3 percent black/African American, and 1 percent other) (Rogers 2014).

Approximately one in four practicing RDNs (23 percent) work part time and/or only part of the year. Seventy-seven percent of RDNs are employed on a full-time basis, defined in the 2013 Compensation and Benefits Survey as being 35 hours or more per week for 48 weeks or more per year. Five percent of RDNs and 2 percent of DTRs report that they are owners or partners in their practices (Rogers 2014).

According to the Commission on Dietetic Registration, as of October 2015, there are 93,946 RD/RDNs in the United States and 5,461 DTRs.

For board certification, there are 895 board certified specialists in pediatric nutrition (CSP), 763 board certified specialists in sports dietetics (CSSD), 693 board certified specialists in oncology nutrition (CSO), 598 board certified specialists in renal nutrition (CSR), and 588 board certified specialist in gerontological nutrition (CSG) (CDR, 2015). An overwhelming majority of credentialed RD/RDNs are white (more than 76,000) and female (94 percent). Almost all RD/RDNs are living or working in the United States, with less than 1,000 located overseas. California has the greatest population of RDNs at 9,883 and Alaska is the least populous state for RDNs with 201.

Compensation

The majority of the data pertaining to compensation for nutrition professionals comes from the Academy of Nutrition and Dietetics' most recent 2013 Compensation and Benefits Survey of the Dietetics Profession. While there are many categories of individuals who can be considered to work in the nutrition profession, this particular survey defined dietetics-related employment as, "A dietetics-related position is considered to be any position that requires or makes use of your education, training, and/or experience in nutrition or dietetics, including situations outside of 'traditional' dietetics practice" (AND, 2013).

There exists a range of information regarding salary of nutrition professionals. The U.S. Bureau of Labor Statistics defines occupational employment and wages for dietitians and nutritionists who "plan and conduct food service or nutritional programs to assist in the promotion of health and control of disease." These individuals "may supervise activities of a department providing quantity food services, counsel individuals, or conduct nutritional research." As of May 2014, the U.S. Bureau of Labor Statistics data indicates that the mean hourly wage in this category is $27.62 and mean annual wage is $57,440. These values reflect a relative standard error in employment of 1.4 percent and 0.4 percent in wages for 59,490 employed individuals (USBLS, 2015).

The AND 2013 Compensation and Benefits Survey provides slightly different wage and salary data—as of April 1, 2013 the median hourly wage was $28.85. When annualized to a 40-hours per week and 52-week per year basis, this equates to a full-time salary of $60,000. This was up 3.5 percent from $27.99 per hour or $58,000 per year in the 2011 survey (Rogers 2014).

Nutrition professionals employed in the practice areas of food and nutrition management, consultation, and business as well as education and research tend to have the highest wages. Wages are lowest for practitioners working in the areas of clinical nutrition-inpatient and community nutrition. By employment sector, those practitioners who are self-employed can expect to earn the highest median hourly wage ($32.45), followed by those who work in government ($29.33). Salaries go down for those working at for-profit ($28.56) or nonprofit institutions ($28.85) (Rogers 2014).

In some regards, the level of education can be correlated with wages earned. The difference between the median wage of an RDN with a bachelor as his or her highest degree (any major) and an RDN with a master's degree (any major) was $1.89 per hour in 2013. Having a PhD is associated with higher earnings as median earnings for those with a doctorate at $36.06 per hour are more than $8 per hour above RDNs who have just a bachelor's degree (Rogers 2014).

The amount of time that one has practiced also contributes to earning potential. Individuals who have been in the field for more than 20 years earn a median wage of more than $9 per hour above those who have been in the field for less than 5 years. An entry-level dietitian can expect to earn $22.60 per hour in 2013, up from $21.63 per hour in 2011 (Rogers 2014). Table 4.4 contains information about hourly wages of RDNs by practice area of primary position. An RDN who has worked in his or her area of practice for more than 10 years can expect to earn over $5 per hour more than those who have been in the position for less than 5 years.

When it comes to acuity level of patient treated, it does not appear that the nutritional risk of the patient treated by the nutrition professional correlates with the earned wages. Median amounts earned are relatively the same for those who work primarily with high-risk patients ($28.37 per hour) compared to those who work mostly with lower-risk patients ($27.88 per hour). At approximately $6 per hour more, RDNs who do not see patients or clients earn substantially higher wages than

Table 4.4 RDN hourly wage by practice area of primary position, from 2013 Compensation and Benefits Survey of the Dietetics Profession (Rogers 2014)

	Number of Respondents	25th Percentile	50th Percentile	75th Percentile
All RDNs	6,048	$24.04	$28.85	$34.86
Inpatient	1,895	$23.08	$26.85	$31.25
Outpatient/ambulatory care	1,042	$24.84	$28.85	$32.98
Long-term care (LTC)	486	$24.04	$28.37	$34.62
Community	715	$21.87	$26.06	$31.25
Food and nutrition management	739	$29.23	$35.58	$43.08
Consultation and business	444	$25.00	$31.54	$40.05
Education and research	360	$24.05	$31.25	$39.26

do those who are involved in direct patient care. The rationale behind this difference is because those who do not see patients or clients are responsible for other tasks that are linked to higher wages, such as serving as faculty members or consultants, being involved in management and supervisory functions, or having budget authority (Rogers 2014).

With regards to benefit packages, the 2013 Compensation and Benefits Survey of the Dietetics Profession found that as a group, dietetics practitioners are offered considerable benefit packages through their employer. Eighty-three percent of respondent say their employers offer some type of retirement package. Eighty-five percent of practitioners are offered some form of paid time off and 73 percent receive one or more of the benefits defined as "professional/career development" which is led by funding and/or time off for professional development as well as college tuition for employees (Rogers 2014).

The Academy of Nutrition and Dietetics has a salary calculator for RDNs available at https://www.eatrightpro.org/resource/career/career-development/salary-calculator/salary-calculator-rdn. This salary calculation worksheet for U.S. RDNs is based on a statistical model developed with data from the Compensation and Benefits Survey of the Dietetics Profession 2013, conducted and analyzed for the Academy of Nutrition and Dietetics by Readex Research. The RDN model was estimated from responses of 4,287 full-time RDNs with an hourly wage in the range of $16.00 to $66.00 (roughly $33,000 to $137,000 annualized) (AND, 2013a).

References

Academy of Nutrition and Dietetics. 2013. *2013 Compensation and Benefits Survey of the Dietetics Profession.* Chicago: Academy of Nutrition and Dietetics.

Academy of Nutrition and Dietetics. 2013a. *Salary Calculator for Registered Dietitian Nutritionists.* www.eatrightpro.org/resource/career/career-development/salary-calculator/salary-calculator-rdn, (accessed October 13, 2015).

Academy of Nutrition and Dietetics. 2015. *Media.* www.eatrightpro.org/resources/media, (accessed October 13, 2015).

Commission on Dietetic Registration. 2015. *Registry Statistics.* www.cdrnet.org/registry-statistics, (accessed October 13, 2015).

Pew Research Center. 2014. *Pew Internet Project's Health Fact Sheet.* www.pewinternet.org/fact-sheets/health-fact-sheet/, (accessed October 13, 2015).

Rogers, D. January, 2014. "Compensation and Benefits Survey 2013: Education and Job Responsibility Key to Increased Compensation." *Journal of the Academy of Nutrition and Dietetics* 114, no. 1, pp. 17–33.

Sports, Cardiovascular and Wellness Nutrition. 2015. *Board Certified Specialist in Sports Dietetics (CSSD).* www.scandpg.org/sports-nutrition/be-a-board-certified-sports-dietitian-cssd/, (accessed October 13, 2015).

US Bureau of Labor Statistics. 2015. *Occupational Employment and Wages, May 2014 29-1031 Dietitians and Nutritionists.* www.bls.gov/oes/current/oes291031.htm#(1), (accessed October 13, 2015).

US Department of Health and Human Services. 2014. *Dietitians.* www.usphs.gov/profession/dietitian/, (accessed October 13, 2015).

US Peace Corps. 2014. *Fact Sheet.* files.peacecorps.gov/multimedia/pdf/about/pc_facts.pdf, (accessed October 13, 2015).

CHAPTER 5

The Future of the Field of Nutrition and Dietetics

Chapter Abstract

Where do we go from here? For individuals currently employed in the field of dietetics or those interested in entering the profession, the future in nutrition is certainly bright. While we have made great advances in the development of evidence-based practice and nutrition science, there is certainly no shortage of a continued need for better eating habits and more active lifestyles in our local and larger communities. With two-thirds of the U.S. population currently overweight or obese and over 90 percent of physicians having never taken a dedicated nutrition course, the need for credentialed nutrition professionals practicing and contributing to the profession is considerable.

The U.S. Bureau of Labor Statistics predicts that employment of dietitians and nutritionists is projected to grow 21 percent from 2012 to 2022, which is faster than the average for all occupations. More dietitians and nutritionists will be needed to meet the growing demands of providing patient care for individuals with a variety of medical conditions and to advise people who want to improve their overall health (USBLS, 2014). This chapter outlines the future of the field of nutrition and dietetics.

Emphasizing Education

In the increasingly noisy landscape of health care in the United States, registered dietitian nutritionists (RDNs) and dietetic technicians, registered (DTRs) increasingly need to differentiate themselves from other nutrition practitioners who may not enter the field with the same rigorous training as them. The core foundations of the RDN and DTR credential include a solid understanding of nutrition science, an ability to implement evidence-based guidelines, and a commitment to provide reliable and consistent care to help promote optimal outcomes. As mentioned in Chapter 3, in 2012 the Academy of Nutrition and Dietetics (AND) proposed to elevate the educational preparation for the future entry-level RDN to a minimum of a graduate degree from an Accreditation Council for Education in Nutrition and Dietetics (ACEND)-accredited program. Currently, the entry-level registration eligibility education requirement is a baccalaureate degree. The recommendation for graduate degree will take place beginning in the year 2024.

There has been much discussion surrounding the future requirement for entry-level practitioners to first obtain a master's degree. Ultimately, the goal is to elevate the level of practice and to push compensation for RDNs to a level commensurate with their professional preparation. Other disciplines outside of nutrition have graduate level requirements for their entry-level practitioners, and one can argue that their higher starting and average salaries may be attributable to their academic achievements and more stringent entry-level education requirements. Those in agreement with the changes in entry-level requirements for dietetics support the new requirements as a means to increase compensation for credentialed nutrition professionals.

In addition to preparatory education for practice, continuing professional education will remain a cornerstone of the RDN/DTR credentials. In the era of Internet diploma mills and self-proclaimed "nutritionist" experts everywhere, the benefit of continuing professional education for legitimately credentialed experts is overwhelming. Nutrition is an evolving science: new discoveries are continuously being made, new research is added to our existing pool of evidence, new (and confusing) food products and supplements flood the product marketplace—all of these provide a continuing opportunity for nutrition professionals to hone their skills and transfer knowledge to an eager and interested patient and client base.

Getting Paid for Services

RDNs are challenged to keep pace with the changing face of health care. With the advent of the Patient Protection and Affordable Care Act (ACA), interest in and access to preventive services has increased for the general public. Millions of Americans can now obtain health insurance through state health exchanges. Nutrition professionals are most concerned about what is ultimately included in the "essential health benefits package," which includes the minimum coverage for individuals who are enrollees in these plans. The Academy of Nutrition and Dietetics advocates for Medical Nutrition Therapy (MNT) provided by an RDN at the federal level through the regulatory process. Getting paid for services rendered by RDNs is essential to the future of the field.

The first step in getting paid for services is proving that those services work. AND's *MNTWorks* campaign aims to highlight the effectiveness—and cost-effectiveness—of medical nutrition therapy provided by a nutrition professional. MNT is linked to improved clinical outcomes and reduced costs related to physician time, medication use and hospital admissions for people with obesity, diabetes and disorders of lipid metabolism along with other chronic diseases (AND, EAL, 2008).

One study showed that prenatal nutrition programs that target high-risk pregnant women have been shown to improve long-term health outcomes in children, saving at least $8 for each dollar invested in the program (Duquette et al. 2008). The Academy provides tools for members to highlight the effectiveness and cost savings of MNT, to negotiate with third-party payers for inclusion of nutrition benefits, to introduce primary care practitioners to the benefits of partnering with RDNs, and to promote an evidence base that shows nutrition as an effective component of comprehensive medical prevention, management, and treatment programs.

Medicare Reimbursement for MNT

Across the nation, health plan and employer coverage of MNT varies. Medicare Part B (Medical Insurance) covers medical nutrition therapy services and certain related services. Since 2002, registered dietitians or nutrition professionals who meet certain requirements can provide

MNT for a limited number of diagnoses and disease states. MNT may include nutritional assessment and one-on-one counseling and therapy services, and this may be done in person or through an interactive tele-communication system. People with Part B who meet at least one of these three conditions are covered for MNT with a qualified nutrition professional who is a Medicare provider:

- Diabetes
- Kidney disease
- Have had a kidney transplant in the last 36 months

Individuals who receive dialysis at a dialysis facility have nutrition coverage provided by Medicare which covers medical nutrition therapy as a part of the overall dialysis care (CMS, 2015).

Reimbursement for Diabetes Treatment

Dietitians are eligible for designation by third-party payers to be eligible providers of MNT and other self-management education and training interventions involved in diabetes care. Medicare includes diabetes as one of the three conditions (as listed above) for which RD/MNT providers may be reimbursed. The *RD Standards of Practice and Standards of Professional Performance for Registered Dietitians (Generalist, Specialty, and Advanced) in Diabetes Care* requires that generalist RDNs be trained to provide MNT and counseling for improved diabetes outcomes. Some RDNs with advanced practice experience may train and test to carry the Certified Diabetes Educator (CDE) credential. The CDE credential identifies individuals like RDs who have experience in diabetes care and education.

Reimbursement for Obesity Treatment

The way we view obesity has changed in recent years. In 2013 the American Medical Association officially recognized obesity as a disease. The direct intent was to induce physicians to give more direct attention to the condition and for insurance companies to begin compensating for treatment. The Internal Revenue Service (IRS) has also ruled that obesity is a disease, meaning that medically-valid weight loss programs are tax-deductible and qualify for new health savings accounts. These changes open up opportunities for RDNs to exert their position as food and nutrition experts in the battle against obesity. AND continues to fight for dietitians' right to bill directly for obesity therapy. Currently, Medicare covers obesity counseling services under the coordination of the primary care provider and makes no direct payments to registered dietitians.

The Academy of Nutrition and Dietetics' Strategic Plan

In 2008 the Academy of Nutrition and Dietetics' Board of Directors activated a new strategic plan and began deliberations on branding the uniqueness of the registered dietitian. The vision of the strategic plan is "Optimizing health through food and nutrition" and the mission is "Empowering members to be food and nutrition leaders." The strategic plan outlines values for the practitioner that include:

- Customer focus—meeting the needs and exceed the expectations of all customers
- Integrity—acting ethically with accountability for lifelong learning, commitment to excellence and professionalism
- Innovation—embracing change with creativity and strategic thinking
- Social responsibility—making decisions with consideration for inclusivity as well as environmental, economic, and social implications
- Diversity—recognizing and respect differences in culture, ethnicity, age, gender, race, creed, religion, sexual orientation, physical ability, politics, and socioeconomic characteristics

The full goals of the strategic plan are outlined in Table 5.1.

Table 5.1 Goals of the Academy of Nutrition and Dietetics' strategic plan (AND, 2015a)

Goal 1: The Public Trusts and Chooses Registered Dietitian Nutritionists as Food, Nutrition and Health Experts

Outcomes and Measures:
- Increases in members' perception of Academy achievement of strategic goals
- Increases in visibility of the Academy to media and consumers via eatright.org and other media outlets (online, print, and broadcast)
- Maintenance or increases in consumer rated credibility of RDNs, NDTRs, and the Academy
- Increases in number of RDN and NDTR appointments to external organizations
- Increases in number of invitations to present Academy initiatives to external medical and other health care disciplines and their organizations

Goal 2: Academy Members Optimize the Health of Individuals and Populations Served

Outcomes and Measures:
- Increases in members' perception of Academy achievement of strategic goals
- Increases in Affiliate Advocacy, Dietetic Practice Group, Academy committee and Academy Employee Engagement Indices
- Increases in level of collaboration (e.g., more engagement) that strengthen relevant partnerships to promote legislative efforts, including more influential partners, members of Congress and federal agencies
- Increases in utilization of the EAL, an Academy member benefit

Goal 3: Members and Prospective Members View the Academy as Vital to Professional Success

Outcomes and Measures:
- Increases in members' perception of Academy achievement of strategic goals
- Increases in Academy membership over time
- Increases in membership market share of nutrition and dietetics practitioners, and students in accredited programs
- Increases in perceived value of Academy membership
- Increases in the diversity of nutrition and dietetics professionals
- Increases in utilization of eatrightPRO.org, an Academy member benefit
- Increases in the number of nutrition and dietetics practitioners
- Increases in enrollment in supervised practice programs

Goal 4: Members Collaborate Across Disciplines with International Food and Nutrition Communities

Outcomes and Measures:
- Increases in members' perception of Academy achievement of strategic goals
- Increases in number of publications and presentations on international initiatives
- Increases in member engagement in international initiatives

- Increases in number of practice resources for international practitioners in collaboration with international nutrition organizations
- Increases in collaborative research with international colleagues
- Increases in number of professional development opportunities for international practitioners in collaboration with other organizations
- Increases in number of government, WHO and UN collaborations

The Academy's Future and You

As a current or future nutrition professional, you are (or will become) a member of a unique group of caring individuals dedicated to improving health outcomes through the provision of food and nutrition education and information. Involvement in your professional organization and associations is essential for the future of the field. As Eldridge Cleaver once paraphrased the Bible, "If you are not a part of the solution, you are a part of the problem" (or in Biblical terms, "Whoever is not with me is against me."). Every member of the nutrition community can find a way to contribute to the greater good of the field. You can volunteer with your local dietetic association, speak to school children about the importance of nutrition, help those in need through work in soup kitchens or food pantries, or teach nutrition classes to a local club or sports team.

To make the goals of the strategic plan come to life, the Academy of Nutrition and Dietetics has *10 Tips to Make the Strategic Plan Your Own*:

1. Understand the critical role you play in both strategy development and strategy implementation.
2. Take a more active role in improving the health of Americans.
3. Review the goals and focus on results you want to achieve.
4. Adapt the values that are specific to your program of work.
5. Integrate your plan into your day-to-day operation.
6. Get and stay connected to the Academy and the strategic plan—read the Daily News, log on to eatrightPRO.org, etc.
7. Once you have adapted the plan, keep your plan alive.
8. Develop specific action steps (tactics) to implement your strategy.
9. Monitor progress of those action steps quarterly.
10. Remember, it's one thing to adapt the Academy's strategic plan and quite another to implement it. Work the plan and make it your own! (AND, 2015)

References

Academy of Nutrition and Dietetics. 2015a. *10 Tips to Make the Strategic Plan Your Own.* www.eatrightpro.org/resource/leadership/board-of-directors/strategic-plan/10-tips-to-make-the-strategic-plan-your-own, (accessed October 15, 2015).

Academy of Nutrition and Dietetics. 2015b. *What Is the Academy's Strategic Plan?* www.eatrightpro.org/resource/leadership/board-of-directors/strategic-plan/what-is-the-academys-strategic-plan, (accessed October 13, 2015).

Academy of Nutrition and Dietetics Evidence Analysis Library. 2008. *Medical Nutrition Therapy Evidence Analysis Project 2008.* www.andeal.org, (accessed October 13, 2015).

Centers for Medicare & Medicaid Services. 2015. *Nutrition Therapy Services (Medical).* www.medicare.gov/coverage/nutrition-therapy-services.html, (accessed October 13, 2015).

Duquette, M.P., H. Payette, J.M. Moutquin, T. Demmers, and J. Desrosiers-Choquette. January, 2008. "Validation of a Screening Tool to Identify the Nutritionally At-risk Pregnancy." *Journal of Obstetrics and Gynaecology Canada* 1, pp. 29–37.

US Bureau of Labor Statistics. 2014. *Dietitians and Nutritionists.* www.bls.gov/ooh/healthcare/dietitians-and-nutritionists.htm, (accessed October 13, 2015).

Index

OTHER TITLES IN OUR NUTRITION AND DIETETIC PRACTICE COLLECTION

Katie Ferraro, *Editor*

- *Diet and Disease: Nutrition for Heart Disease, Diabetes and Metabolic Stress Nutrition for Heart Disease, Diabetes, and Metabolic Stress* by Katie Ferraro
- *Diet and Disease: Nutrition for Gastrointestinal, Musculoskeletal, Hepatobiliary, Pancreatic, and Kidney Diseases* by Katie Ferraro
- *Nutrition Support* by Brenda O'Day
- *Weight Management and Obesity* by Courtney Winston Paolicelli

Momentum Press is one of the leading book publishers in the field of engineering, mathematics, health, and applied sciences. Momentum Press offers over 30 collections, including Aerospace, Biomedical, Civil, Environmental, Nanomaterials, Geotechnical, and many others.

Momentum Press is actively seeking collection editors as well as authors. For more information about becoming an MP author or collection editor, please visit http://www.momentumpress.net/contact

Announcing Digital Content Crafted by Librarians

Momentum Press offers digital content as authoritative treatments of advanced engineering topics by leaders in their field. Hosted on ebrary, MP provides practitioners, researchers, faculty, and students in engineering, science, and industry with innovative electronic content in sensors and controls engineering, advanced energy engineering, manufacturing, and materials science.

Momentum Press offers library-friendly terms:
- perpetual access for a one-time fee
- no subscriptions or access fees required
- unlimited concurrent usage permitted
- downloadable PDFs provided
- free MARC records included
- free trials

The **Momentum Press** digital library is very affordable, with no obligation to buy in future years.

For more information, please visit **www.momentumpress.net/library** or to set up a trial in the US, please contact **mpsales@globalepress.com**.

www.ingramcontent.com/pod-product-compliance
Lightning Source LLC
Chambersburg PA
CBHW061609220326
41598CB00024BC/3517